eventive
Medicine

Natural Options for Keeping Well

PREVENTIVE MEDICINE

Created, edited, and designed by
Quadrille Publishing Limited

© 1996 Quadrille Publishing
All rights reserved. Unauthorized reproduction, in
any manner, is prohibited.

TIME
LIFE
BOOKS

TIME-LIFE BOOKS
Staff for Preventive Medicine
Editorial Manager Christine Noble
Design Director Mary Staples
Cover Design Nina Bridges
Cover Photograph Marie Claire Idees: Yoichiro Sato,
Martine Paillard
Editorial Production Justina Cox

American Adaptation Heather Ostrem Lyons,
Tina McDowell, Miriam Newton, Barbara Fairchild
Quarmby, Janet Syring, Marlene Zack

Library of Congress Cataloging in Publication Data
Preventive medicine: natural options for keeping well/
  by the editors of Time-Life Books.
      p.   cm.
    Includes bibliographical references and index.
    ISBN 0-7835-4916-4
    I. Self-care, Health.   2. Medicine, Preventive—
Popular works.   3. Holistic medicine.
I. Time-Life Books.
RA776.95.P74   1997
613--dc20   96-43447
                         CIP

QUADRILLE PUBLISHING
Publishing Director Anne Furniss
Project Editor Clare Hill
Editors Mary Lambert, Jon Kirkwood, Jerome Burne
Art Director Mary Evans
Art Editor Alison Fenton
Designers Jo Tapper, Sue Rawkins, Vanessa Courtier
Editorial Assistant Katherine Seely

CONTRIBUTORS
Planning, Research, and Text Lisha Simester
Fitness Plans Joanna Berry
Special Photography Sandra Lousada, Carl Warner
Illustrations Alison Barrett, Lucy Su, Julia Whatley

CONSULTANTS
Series Consultant Lisha Simester
Kenneth Kahn PhD, MD, MIBiol.
Rodney Adeniyi-Jones MRCP (U.K.)
Pierre-Jean Cousin MBACC, GCRCH (Acupuncture
    and Chinese Herbalism)
Max Deacon MB, BS, MF Hom. (Homeopathy)
Caroline Peters ITEC, AIPTI (Reflexology)
Germaine Rich MIFA (Aromatherapy)
Claerwen Williams MA (Psychotherapy)
Eddie and Debbie Shapiro (Meditation and
    Relaxation)
Karen Kingston (Feng Shui)

The textual and visual descriptions of medical
conditions and treatment options in this book
should be considered as a reference source only;
they are not intended to substitute for a healthcare practitioner's diagnosis, advice, and treatment.
Always consult your physician or a qualified practitioner for proper medical care.

TIME-LIFE is a trademark of Time Warner Inc. U.S.A.

TIME-LIFE BOOKS is a division of Time Life Inc.

Preventive Medicine

Natural Options for Keeping Well

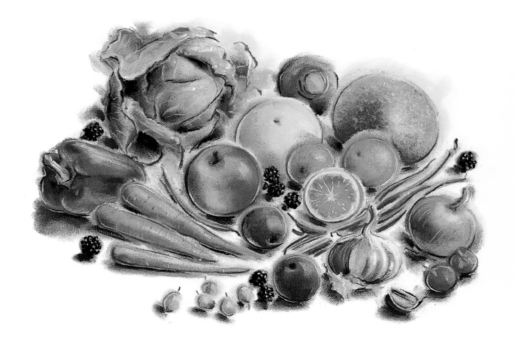

Time-Life Books, Alexandria, Virginia

CONTENTS

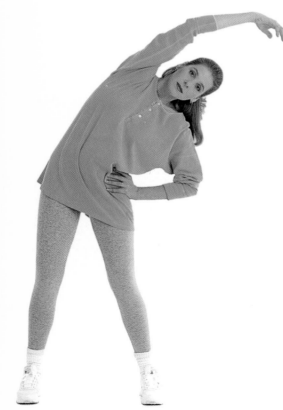

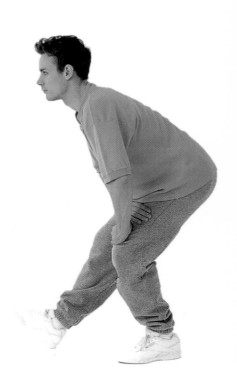

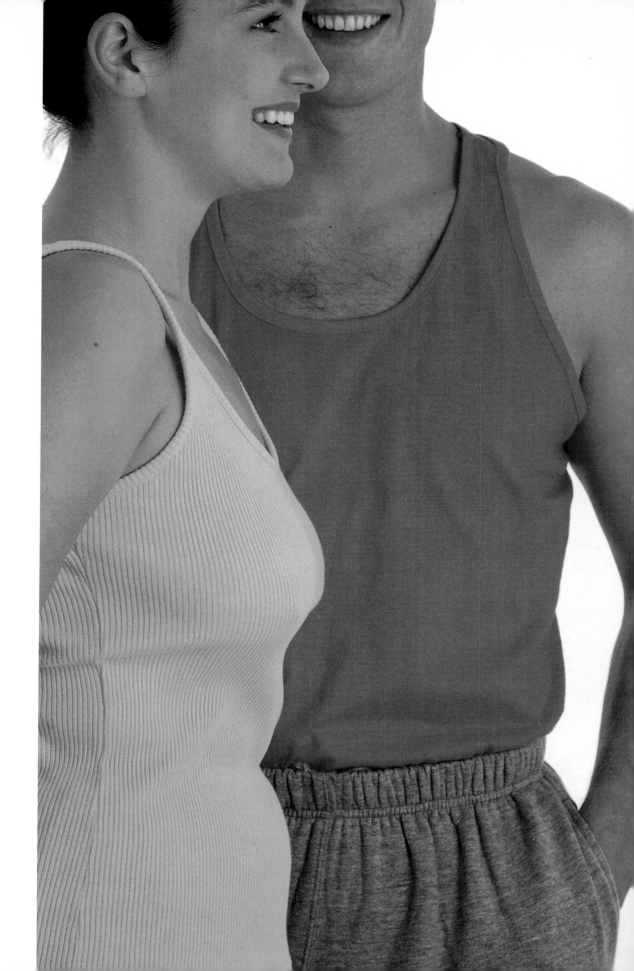

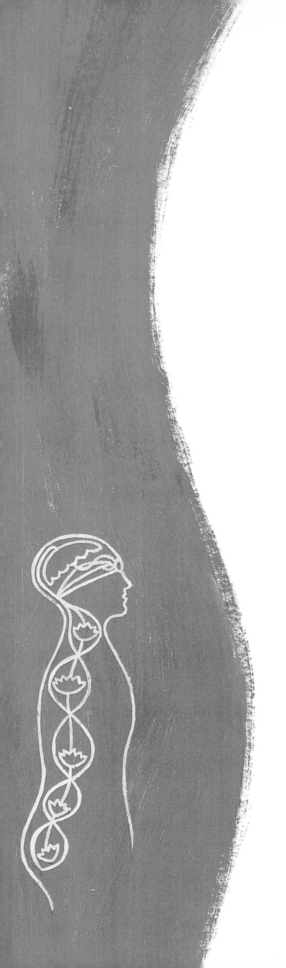

I
The Well Body

What is a well body and what are the systems working within us that hold the key to our well-being? Understanding how the parts add up to a whole body and how we can create optimum well-being through a balanced, holistic approach to our health is our goal in this chapter.

Health and well-being are an individual and unique experience—there cannot be one rule for all. Holistic medicine looks at the whole person, taking into account diet and lifestyle, before attempting to evaluate the condition of body and mind.

To reach a level of whole health and well-being we must realize that as individuals, we have the ability to achieve an optimum level of health and a balanced body and mind by reviewing our health habits honestly and implementing a few simple lifestyle changes. Glowing good health is within our reach if we make the right choices about the way we live.

How Well Are You?

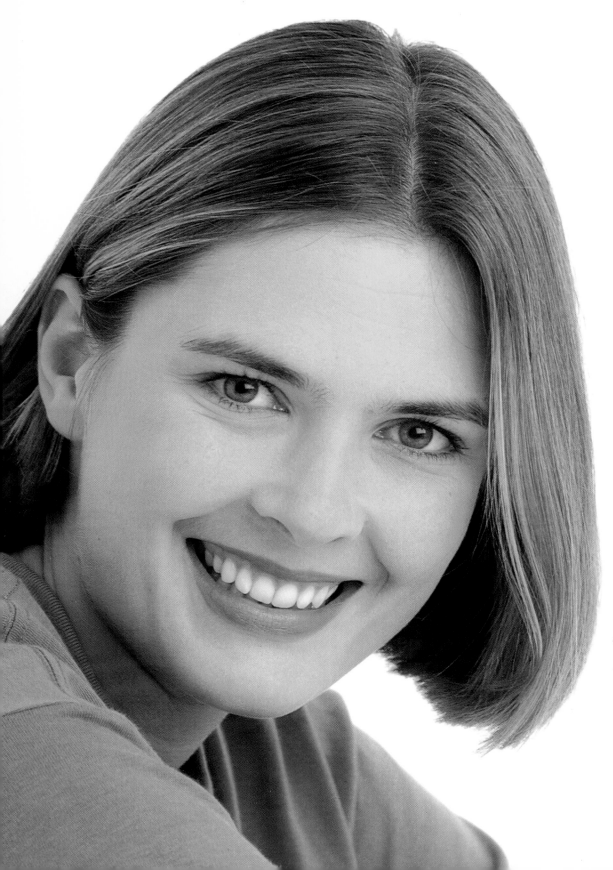

The healthy body has a glowing look, bright eyes, clear skin, and shiny hair. By eating well, exercising, relaxing, and knowing how to combat stress you can achieve a much greater state of well-being and—above all—a greater zest for life.

Assess your well-being

Our bodies have a way of letting us know what they need. A knot in the stomach may not be indigestion but may be caused by stress. Feeling lethargic could mean that we need to change our diet. Lower-back pain could be telling us to change the way we sit or stand. A scaly skin could mean it is time to take a vitamin supplement. Unless we pick up on these signs we might miss an important message—a message that our health is in danger. But there is much more to overall well-being than dealing with illness. If you know what to look for in your body and mind then you can recognize the signals that can tell you what improvements to make to optimize your health.

Most people would agree that a well body is one that is free of serious imbalances, excesses, toxins, and dysfunction, and certainly free from degenerative disease. To reach a level of whole health and well-being we have to take responsibility for our health and create a personalized system of preventive measures. This can often be done by implementing a few basic lifestyle changes. As a start toward an honest review of your health habits, take a look at the questions and answers on the right.

Q. Why do I need to know all about how my body works?

Without accurate and appropriate information about the way your body works, its needs and the best strategies for optimum health, you cannot really choose how to live your life to ensure you keep well. If you know how your body does its job, what the threats are to its well-being, and exactly what you can do to keep it healthy, then you are doing very well. And if you are actually acting upon this information, you should be healthy.
(See the following pages in this chapter.)

Q. Does the food I eat really make a difference to my well-being?

While you can get by eating anything for a while, a proper appreciation of the benefits of a good diet is essential if you are to eat what you need to feel at your best. By taking the right foodstuffs at the right time you can not only avoid potential problems but give your health and energy levels a dramatic boost. Food has, in fact, been called the miracle medicine. Can you take a balanced view about a balanced diet?
(See Chapter 2.)

Q. The claims made about dietary supplements are baffling. How can I tell if I need anything extra in my diet?

There are definitely times when taking a dietary supplement of some vitamins or minerals is a good idea, if not essential. But just as important is knowing what *not* to take, or when a dose is dangerous. Do you know all the signs that tell you when it is the right time to take a supplement?
(See Chapter 3.)

Q. What are the therapies that can help me to prevent disease and illness?

Conventional and alternative medicine can be combined to make a powerful shield against the ailments that can make you feel bad and make you more susceptible to illness. Knowledge about a range of alternative therapies allows you to select what may be right for you. Can you say you have considered all the possibilities available?
(See Chapter 4.)

Q. We all know that exercise is good for us but how do I plan an activity schedule that fits in with my needs?

Many people exercise the wrong way and this puts undue strain on their bodies, leading to injury. Of course this will discourage you from exercising! Also, choosing a form of exercise that is difficult from a practical point of view, requiring lots of traveling or expensive equipment, may also deter you. Do you really know the right type of exercise for you and how to make it an enjoyable, indispensable part of your life?
(See Chapter 5.)

Q. So many people seem unable to deal with this unfriendly modern world. How can I cope with the pressures of living today?

There is so much more to life than simply avoiding feeling bad. Stress can be dealt with, you can change your life for the better, you can discover ways to know more about the real you, and the pursuit of happiness need not be fruitless. If you are mentally strong a crisis can be handled better and you can give help to others in their times of need. Can you truthfully say there is nothing in your mind that needs tackling?
(See Chapter 6.)

Q. Is it really necessary for me to take time out to unwind?

Proper relaxation techniques and long-term stress-management methods can assist you in feeling calm and in control. There are some things you can do that will recharge and regenerate your mind and body. Have you found out how to let go of negative thoughts and emotions and energize your whole being?
(See Chapter 7.)

Life Transitions

From childhood to old age many biological changes take place in the body. Knowing about them allows us to make decisions that will help us achieve optimum good health and happiness. It is important to recognize the different needs we have at different times and to prepare for these various transitions.

In infancy and childhood our well-being is almost entirely dependent on the wisdom and knowledge of parents and teachers. Parents make sure we eat well and regularly, keep us clean and washed, and make sure we go to bed early enough to get the vital sleep our growing bodies and minds require. It is never too early for parents and teachers to encourage a child to adopt healthy ways of living since the health habits of a lifetime begin in childhood. For instance, children are strongly attracted to sweets and junk food, but they can be taught that healthier, natural snacks, such as fruit, are just as good. If children are allowed to watch too much television or play at the computer for too long, then couch potato habits could set in. In many children a lack of regular exercise becomes a habit that they take with them into adulthood, minimizing their chances for healthy, strong bodies that can achieve and maintain optimum health throughout life.

Whatever stage of life you are in, however, there are many things you can do to enhance your life and health. And even if you do have ingrained, unhealthy habits, it is never too late to change.

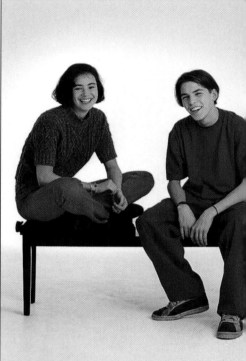

Adolescence

During puberty, dramatic hormonal changes take place. Girls become young women and boys young men, at least sexually. Puberty is triggered by the brain's pituitary gland, which controls the flow of sex hormones. These in turn bring on the development of the sex organs and the other physical changes that come with maturity. Both body and mind are changing and this can be a very confusing and emotional time.

• Adolescents need to eat food rich in calcium because the bones are growing so quickly. Encourage them to eat more fruits and vegetables and try to limit their intake of junk food.
• Encourage sports and exercise.
• Adolescents are painfully aware of their looks and hormonal changes can cause problems such as acne, oily skin, and limp, dull, or dry hair. Encourage them to take care of their appearance.

20s–30s

These are the years when youth is still on our side and we should maintain or begin a healthy lifestyle that can both prevent later degenerative disease and delay the effects of aging. Since these are the years when most people start families, it is vital to make sure you eat healthy, wholesome food.

• Start eating low-fat foods and taking cod liver oil and flaxseed oil supplements to help prevent fatty deposits in your arteries.
• Exercise regularly.
• Eat lots of fresh fruits and vegetables.
• Learn relaxation techniques to alleviate the stress that working life brings.
• Women planning pregnancy should eat more deep green and leafy vegetables, particularly broccoli, and take folic acid supplements three months prior to anticipated conception and three months after conception. Folic acid may help prevent spina bifida and other birth defects.

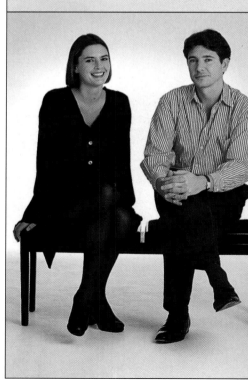

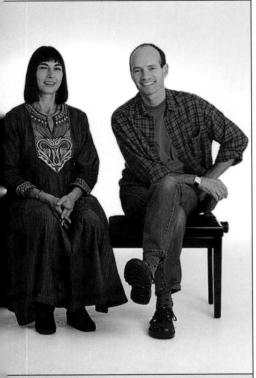

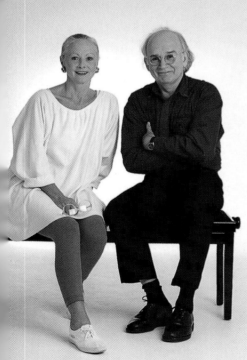

40s–50s

This is a time of real change, when our bodies begin to show signs of aging. Hair begins to go gray, some people gain weight, particularly around the middle, skin loses some of its elasticity, and wrinkles can deepen. If you want to stay healthy and prevent illness you must take extra care of your body *now*. For women a good diet and regular exercise will help during menopause. This time usually lasts three to four years, the few years before your last period and the year after, when hormone levels drop. Exercise and proper eating are important for men, too, who are entering the high-risk category for heart disease.

- If you have not already started, this is the time to implement a regular exercise program to ensure mobility in later years. If in any doubt about your health, and especially before starting a strenuous regimen, consult your family doctor.
- Eat foods high in protective vitamins—fruit and yellow and leafy green vegetables.
- Eat foods high in calcium and magnesium to prevent osteoporosis.
- In your 50s your body does not need as much food as before, so you can cut back on fat, carbohydrates, and the size of portions.
- Osteoarthritis can be prevented with regular exercise such as walking, swimming, and yoga. Eating oily fish and foods containing selenium (whole grains, asparagus, eggs, garlic, mushrooms) may also help. Consult your healthcare provider before taking selenium supplements.
- Menopausal women can seek alternative treatment to Hormone Replacement Therapy (HRT). Both acupuncture and homeopathy can help. Geranium oil is said to be a hormonal balancer; use during massage or add to the bath.
- Men should have prostate gland exams in their 50s to detect any disorders such as enlargement, inflammation, or cancer.
- Women should begin regular mammograms in their 50s.

Aging

The later decades of life are a time when we reach the high plateau of life. It is a time for reflection and a chance to pass on the experience and wisdom we have gained. To enjoy life to the fullest during this time, healthy eating practices and staying fit and active are even more important. It is a time for positive thinking and new beginnings. The change from a busy working life to one of retirement is a challenge, but retirement should not mean withdrawal from the world; it is a time to develop new interests or get back in touch with things that you always wanted to do but never had the time for.

- Dietary needs change as we get older but we still need to watch the amount of fat we eat and include plenty of fresh fruits and vegetables in our diet.
- Continue to exercise. Swimming is very beneficial and a walk every day helps with circulation and breathing. Yoga or tai chi will help maintain flexibility without putting the joints under stress.
- Keep busy. Explore a new hobby or interest; get involved with volunteer or community groups.
- Become more politically active, as you may have more time to spend on local or national issues.
- Some hearing loss is normal in older people but hearing can be preserved for longer if you protect your ears from loud noises.
- Have regular eye checkups. Falls, which are quite common in older people, often result from an impaired sense of balance and bad eyesight.
- Refuse to conform to ageism. Do what makes you feel happy and fulfilled.

Heart and Circulation

One of the most extraordinary components of the body is its central pumping station—the heart. The healthy heart is an extremely sophisticated machine, beating steadily and unobtrusively somewhere between 60 and 100 times every minute. The heart circulates the average adult's approximately five quarts of blood through about 60,000 miles of blood vessels between 3,000 and 5,000 times every day. By the end of an average lifetime, the heart will have pumped more than 60 million gallons of blood. Such astonishing statistics would put most man-made devices to shame. All this incredible performance and reliability comes from a muscle that weighs between 11 and 16 ounces and is about the size of two clenched fists.

Eat to your heart's content

There are some foods that help protect against heart disease. As much as possible these should be included in your daily diet:
- Raw garlic and onions.
- Oat bran.
- Oatmeal.
- Cooked dried beans.
- Avocados.
- Olive oil.
- Oily fish, such as salmon, herring, sardines, tuna, and mackerel.
- Leafy green and yellow vegetables.
- Fresh fruits.

Avoid refined, highly processed foods, which are often full of fat and sugar, and foods with high levels of animal fat. For some people excess salt can raise blood pressure, which is another risk factor for heart disease. Other foods to avoid include:
- Hydrogenated vegetable oils (solid shortening).
- Refined (white) flour products.

Positive changes that you can make to your diet include:
- Using low-fat dairy products such as skim milk and low-fat cottage cheese. Use a low-fat spread or a margarine that is high in polyunsaturates.
- Reducing your intake of sugar, salt, and alcohol, as well as processed foods, which contain added sugar and salt.
- Eating more oily fish such as salmon, herring, sardines, and mackerel.
- Eating fiber-rich foods such as whole-grain breads, oats, beans, and baked potatoes.
- Eating three to five servings of vegetables and two to four servings of fruit daily.

The heart

At each heartbeat the heart muscle contracts, squeezing the blood within its chambers and forcing it to move under pressure along the blood vessels.

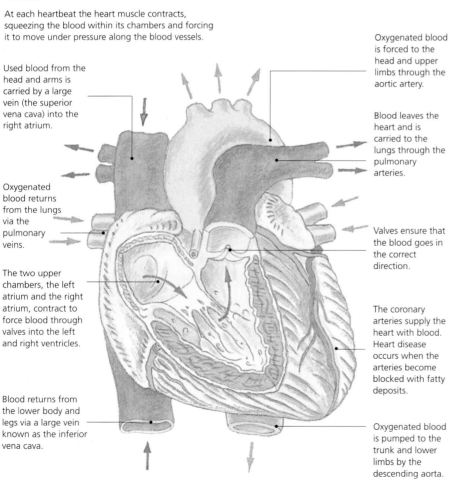

Used blood from the head and arms is carried by a large vein (the superior vena cava) into the right atrium.

Oxygenated blood returns from the lungs via the pulmonary veins.

The two upper chambers, the left atrium and the right atrium, contract to force blood through valves into the left and right ventricles.

Blood returns from the lower body and legs via a large vein known as the inferior vena cava.

Oxygenated blood is forced to the head and upper limbs through the aortic artery.

Blood leaves the heart and is carried to the lungs through the pulmonary arteries.

Valves ensure that the blood goes in the correct direction.

The coronary arteries supply the heart with blood. Heart disease occurs when the arteries become blocked with fatty deposits.

Oxygenated blood is pumped to the trunk and lower limbs by the descending aorta.

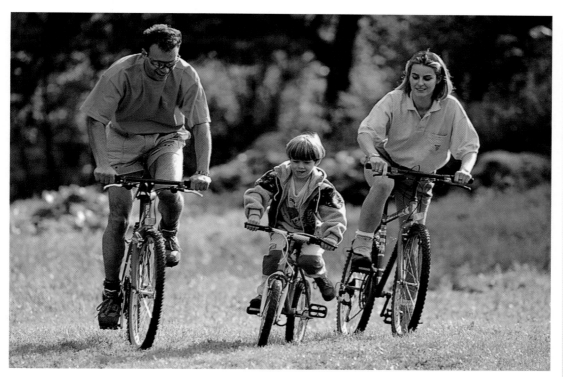

Exercise is very important for maintaining a healthy heart. The heart is a muscle, and like any muscle, it gets stronger with exercise. Try to to do some form of energetic exercise at least every other day. A brisk walk, cycling, swimming, dancing, or any other exercise that increases the heart rate will provide excellent exercise. Exercise can also help in weight loss and can help to lower blood pressure. If you are not fit, and if there is any likelihood that you might have heart disease or high blood pressure, consult a doctor before undertaking exercise.

All living tissue needs a constant flow of blood to function and this is supplied by the heart. One of the blood's key roles is to deliver oxygen to the tissues and take away carbon dioxide. Blood also carries nutrients such as glucose. Without blood the tissues would die. Any problem with the heart is therefore potentially serious and heart disease has become one of the greatest health challenges facing us today.

The most common type of heart disease occurs when the blood vessels supplying the heart become narrowed. A narrowed coronary artery can cause the intermittent pains of angina; a totally blocked artery causes a heart attack. Narrowed arteries occur when the arteries get clogged with fatty deposits, or atheroma. This depositing of plaque in the arteries, known as atherosclerosis, has a number of causes.

There can be an inherited predisposition toward heart disease, and the condition is more likely if a person is overweight, has high blood pressure, exercises too little, smokes, or reacts badly to stress. It can also result from eating too much fat, especially saturated fat (the kind found in meat and dairy products).

Heart disease is unusual before people reach their mid-40s, but men are more prone to it than women at any age. However, many would be surprised to know that the latest statistics show heart disease is the No. 1 cause of death in U.S. women.

Tips for a healthy heart

Heart disease is closely linked to a poor diet and lifestyle. If we adopt a healthier way of living we significantly reduce the risk. Take control of the following factors in your life:

• Don't smoke. It is the single most important contributory factor in heart disease.

• Exercise regularly.

• If you are overweight go on a weight-reducing program.

• Reduce your stress levels—learn how to relax. Take yoga classes or try meditation. Aromatherapy treatment is a great stress reliever.

• Eat a healthy low-fat diet. This means no more than 10 percent of fat in your total food intake.

• Watch your blood cholesterol and blood pressure levels. Follow the advice recommended by your doctor to reduce the levels if they are too high.

The Breath of Life

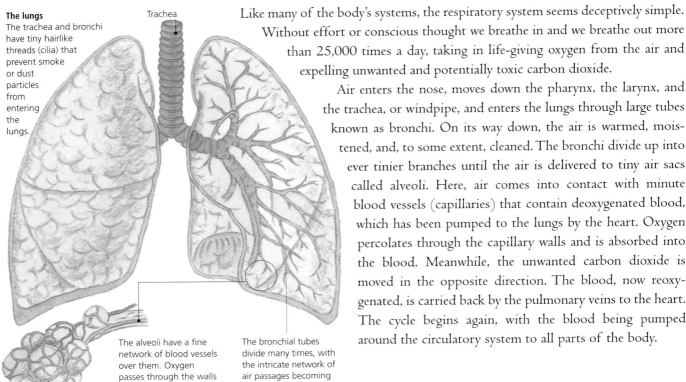

The lungs
The trachea and bronchi have tiny hairlike threads (cilia) that prevent smoke or dust particles from entering the lungs.

Trachea

The alveoli have a fine network of blood vessels over them. Oxygen passes through the walls of the alveoli and into the bloodstream.

The bronchial tubes divide many times, with the intricate network of air passages becoming thinner and thinner at each division.

Like many of the body's systems, the respiratory system seems deceptively simple. Without effort or conscious thought we breathe in and we breathe out more than 25,000 times a day, taking in life-giving oxygen from the air and expelling unwanted and potentially toxic carbon dioxide.

Air enters the nose, moves down the pharynx, the larynx, and the trachea, or windpipe, and enters the lungs through large tubes known as bronchi. On its way down, the air is warmed, moistened, and, to some extent, cleaned. The bronchi divide up into ever tinier branches until the air is delivered to tiny air sacs called alveoli. Here, air comes into contact with minute blood vessels (capillaries) that contain deoxygenated blood, which has been pumped to the lungs by the heart. Oxygen percolates through the capillary walls and is absorbed into the blood. Meanwhile, the unwanted carbon dioxide is moved in the opposite direction. The blood, now reoxygenated, is carried back by the pulmonary veins to the heart. The cycle begins again, with the blood being pumped around the circulatory system to all parts of the body.

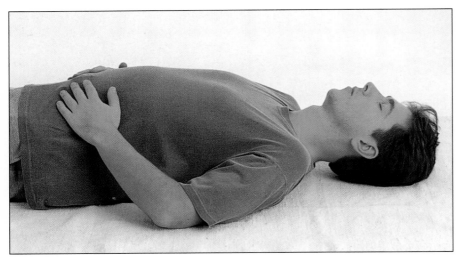

To deep breathe, lie down and place your palms on each side of your abdomen and follow your breath from your nose down through your chest, to your abdomen, and then back. As you inhale, allow the chest and then the abdomen to expand. Exhale, allowing the gentle contraction of first the abdomen and then the chest.

Breathing for good health

In the Western world most people are unaware of the importance that breathing plays in achieving good health and a true state of well-being. We only consider our lungs and the whole subject of breath when breathing becomes a problem, either because of pollution, an allergy such as hay fever, or a degenerative disease of the lungs.

Most of us do not effectively use our respiratory system. We shallow breathe or breathe through the mouth, a method which does not allow enough oxygen into the body. Steady deep breathing not only ensures that the respiratory system is working at peak efficiency but can also have a calming effect on the way we feel. Deep breathing involves

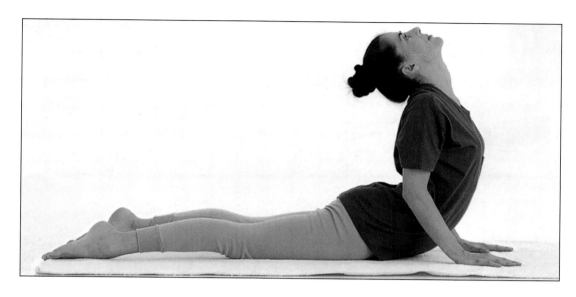

The yogic cobra position shown above involves stretching back to expand the lungs and rib cage. This allows a greater amount of oxygen to enter the lungs and promotes better breathing techniques.

using the diaphragm and abdomen much more fully. Harnessing the power of the lungs with deep-breathing exercises will help you maximize the amount of oxygen in your body, improving posture at the same time.

Health professionals today have joined holistic practitioners in recognizing the importance of breathing in maintaining true well-being. Good breathing habits can relieve the symptoms of many conditions such as asthma, bronchitis, heart disease, chronic fatigue, anxiety, stress, and depression. Breathing well has a dramatic psychological effect. The reason most people say "take a deep breath and let it all out" to someone in deep shock and distress is because we instinctively know that to take a deep breath will help calm the individual or the situation.

Many Eastern mystics have used breathing to control pain and this technique also has a modern application. Controlled breathing helps women in childbirth alleviate their labor pains.

Controlling asthma

Throughout the world, asthma, especially childhood asthma, is increasing dramatically. Opinion is divided as to why asthma rates are rising. Some experts believe environmental factors are to blame. These include pollution (especially from vehicle exhaust), smoking, and home decoration that encourages allergens like dust mites. Others believe that diet, genes, and stress are chiefly responsible. And it seems that there is no escape from asthma—it is as common in the countryside as it is in the cities. Many young children grow out of asthma, but some people suffer throughout life. Asthma sufferers must be under a doctor's care, and they should always have access to an inhaler to prevent or control an attack.

There are various things asthma sufferers can do to improve their condition and their environment. Allergens, such as grass and other pollens, can trigger attacks, as can food allergies. People with asthma soon learn about their own sensitivities and triggers and should be alert to avoiding or controlling them.

Once the early symptoms of an attack begin, find a comfortable sitting or semireclining position. Try to breathe in from the abdomen, using your diaphragm. Breathe out slowly and deliberately. Repeat until you feel better.

Asthma tips

You can help to prevent asthma attacks by following some of these hints:

• Use natural flooring such as wood or tiles instead of wall-to-wall carpets.

• Cut down on central heating and make sure rooms are well ventilated.

• Avoid tobacco smoke in the house.

• Control house dust levels with regular vacuuming and dusting.

• Avoid feather pillows and comforters, anything made of animal fur, and family pets.

• Avoid stressful situations and learn to recognize, manage, and minimize stress.

• If you suffer from asthma, always, always carry your inhaler with you, being careful to use it only as your physician prescribes.

Brain, Nerves, and Glands

The brain and nervous system form the command and communications network of the body, receiving messages from the senses, processing them, and directing and coordinating all actions. They work together with the glands of the endocrine system, which govern the body's hormones, to form a regulation and control system of exquisite refinement and awesome power.

The brain is the home of our thoughts, memories, feelings, talents, perceptions, creative imagination, and inspiration, as well as the initiator and regulator of all our physical, mental, emotional, and spiritual functions. It is, in fact, the most complicated device known to man, despite weighing little more than three pounds.

The brain never shuts down. Even when we are asleep it is still processing information from our five senses. Its central nervous system is made up of over 100 billion tiny nerve cells called neurons. Each neuron is connected to perhaps 10,000 other neurons and they constantly send messages to one another. This activity takes a lot of energy and demands a high level of the body's primary fuel, glucose.

Almost every structure in the brain has its mirror image. Thus there are two cerebral hemispheres and two sides to the cerebellum. Generally, each side deals with the opposite side of the body. The part of the cortex that handles touch messages from the right side of the body is on the left side of the brain. Some of the higher functions are not dealt with in this symmetrical way. For instance, in most people one cerebral hemisphere will handle speech, reading, talking, and logical activities while the other will handle emotional, visual, and spatial functions. Usually, right-handed people have their speech and linked functions dealt with by the left hemisphere, but this is reversed in left-handed people.

Avoiding headaches

Headaches are caused by the tension or stretching of the meninges, the membranes around the brain, or from tension or stretching of the scalp and its blood vessels and muscles.

Certain foods, such as red wine, cheese, and chocolate, are known to trigger headaches, particularly migraines, so avoid eating these foods if they have this effect. Eating regularly helps avoid headaches, as hunger is also a headache trigger.

Hangovers are a well-known cause of headaches and the only way of avoiding them is to limit alcohol intake. Poor posture or stress can cause tension in the neck and shoulders that can manifest itself in headaches, so try to control these factors. Working or living in badly ventilated rooms can cause headaches, so throw open the windows. Gentle exercise, such as walking, keeps the blood flowing properly to all parts of the brain. Try to walk reasonably vigorously for about 20 minutes every day.

Tension headaches can be alleviated with aromatherapy massage while persistent headaches can be successfully treated with acupuncture, which aims to help unblock the energy in the yang channel of the head. Cranial osteopathy and homeopathy treatments have also achieved success in eliminating or controlling debilitating headaches.

The brain

The cortex covers the brain. This is where most of the higher functions—speech, memory, perception, and consciousness—reside.

Touch and muscle control are controlled by two regions of the cerebrum.

The frontal lobe of the cerebrum deals with planning and complex functions, such as personality and the power of abstract thinking.

Speech is dealt with by areas in the temporal lobe of the cerebrum.

The hypothalamus, which is part of the endocrine system, monitors the body's water balance, temperature, hunger, and thirst.

Deep inside the brain is the thalamus, which acts as a relay station for incoming sensory information, and the basal ganglia, which help in controlling movement.

The occipital lobe, or back of the cerebrum, deals with vision.

The cerebellum helps control fine, rapid movements, especially those guided by the senses.

The brainstem deals with many functions including level of arousal, rate of breathing, and the force and rapidity of the heartbeat.

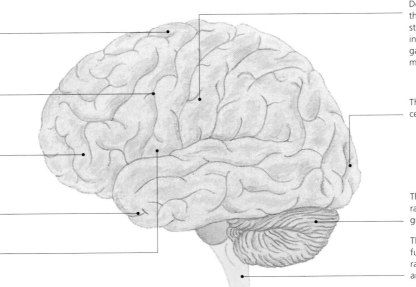

The endocrine glands

The endocrine glands are powerful yet subtle; they determine the nature and efficiency of our entire body chemistry. They are the main regulators of our body's metabolism and they exert their influence by releasing hormones. The endocrine glands are a series of ductless glands that pour the hormones directly into the bloodstream. These glands are located in the central nervous system and in the circulatory, digestive, and reproductive systems.

The central nervous system

The central nervous system, comprising the brain and spinal cord, presides over a map of nerves that run throughout the body carrying electro-chemical messages from the body to the brain, and vice versa. These messages travel extremely quickly—it takes only a fraction of a second for a message to go from the foot all the way to the brain. The nervous system is responsible for all those body actions that we are not in conscious control of, including heart rate, speed of digestion, and contraction of the iris in the eye. It also reacts to life-threatening danger. It commands the adrenal gland to pump out adrenalin, which gets the body ready for emergency action.

Nervous system foods

There are a number of foodstuffs that some experts believe play a part in the healthy functioning of the brain. Following the correct diet—rich in fresh fruits and vegetables and high in complex carbohydrates such as rice, pasta, potatoes, and bread—will give the nervous system the nourishment it requires to function well. Carbohydrates in particular provide the steady supply of the energy sugar, glucose, that the brain needs.

About 20 percent of our brain tissue is made up of lecithin, which is found in soybeans and egg yolks. By eating lecithin in combination with vitamin C and raw garlic you might help clean away cholesterol deposits in the coronary arteries and blood vessels, thereby increasing the blood supply to the brain.

Endocrine and nervous systems

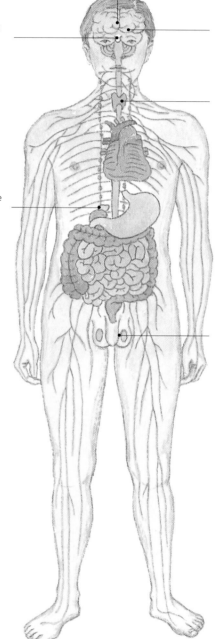

The pituitary is the most important gland in the body and it makes hormones that control most of the other glands, including the growth hormones and those that control the main male and female hormones.

The hypothalamus makes hormones that control certain functions of the pituitary gland.

The brain and spinal cord make up the central nervous system.

The thyroid makes hormones that control the metabolic rate of the body (the rate at which it uses energy).

The adrenal glands produce adrenalin, the fight-or-flight hormone.

The sex glands (testes in men, ovaries in women) make hormones that regulate sexual functions.

Spine, Bones, and Muscles

The central structural component of the human body is the spine. It provides a supportive pillar to the body and is also a protective cover for the spinal cord, the body's primary conduit of nerves, which runs from the base of the skull to the lumbar region of the back. The spine—also called the spinal column—is made up of 26 articulated bones, part of a system of 33 small bones called vertebrae. These are held together and supported by muscles and sheets or bands of fibrous tissue known as ligaments. Most of the vertebrae are separated by disks of particularly tough fibrous tissue that act as protective shock absorbers.

Possessing a spinal column with vertebrae capable of a turning movement distinguishes higher animals from the rest of the animal world. As humans evolved we gradually stopped walking on all fours and became the only species to stand absolutely erect. This has many advantages; but we also pay a price for our upright posture. The excess strain and pressure placed on the spine through standing upright contributes greatly to back problems. Approximately 80 percent of the population is afflicted with backache, either occasionally or on a regular basis.

Most back pain is caused by weakness in the muscles and ligaments. As we grow older, the ligaments become tighter and shorter, causing the backbone to stiffen. This impairs our movements and causes tears in the muscles and ligaments when they are stretched. But this does not have to happen. We can maintain muscle and ligament elasticity with a regular exercise and stretching program. Those who exercise regularly are much less likely to suffer from back pain. In contrast, an inactive lifestyle contributes considerably to weak muscles and thus poorly supported and injury-prone spines. As well as muscle and ligament pain, back pain can occur when there is a problem with an intervertebral disk. If a disk gets out of shape, either as a result of injury or by being put under too much pressure, it can press on a nerve as it leaves the spinal cord. This can cause pain locally or in the region that the nerve travels to. The spine can also be a barometer of our stress levels and emotional state. People who are feeling down, especially men, are more likely to suffer from lower-back pain. Thus it is important to try to deal with emotional problems and to learn how to manage everyday stresses.

Spinal mobility and ligament flexibility play a major role in yogic postures. Yoga teachers believe the key to a healthy and long life is in a pliable spine, so much attention is given to promoting flexibility in the spinal column and its ligaments.

The spine

Seven cervical vertebrae (neck bones) at the top of the spine support the skull.

Twelve thoracic vertebrae make up the longest section of the spine. Each one is attached to a pair of ribs.

Cross section of spinal cord

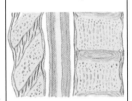

Thirty-one paired nerves carry messages from the body to and from the spinal cord. Nerves emerge along the entire length of the spinal cord, which runs down the center of the spine and acts as an information superhighway, connecting the brain to the body.

The lumbar section contains five vertebrae. They carry the weight of the body above and are vulnerable to damage from lifting heavy loads.

A tough disk of tissue acts as a lubricating joint and shock absorber between all vertebrae that move.

Five fused vertebrae make up the sacrum, which is joined to the pelvis.

The lowest part of the spine is the coccyx, which is made up of four fused vertebrae.

Strengthening the back

Strengthening the back muscles can help avoid back injury or pain and make chronic back conditions less likely to recur. As an added bonus, toned-up muscles will improve both back flexibility and mobility and can also help improve your posture.

The following exercises will help increase spine flexibility and tone the back muscles. They are also good warm-up exercises to do prior to other sports or exercise programs.

If at any point during these exercises you feel any pain, dizziness, or breathing difficulties—stop. Before you try the exercises again you should consult your doctor.

Knee hug and roll
This exercise gently stretches the lower back. Sit on the floor and draw your knees to your chest, hold on to your feet or ankles with your hands. Drop your chin down to your chest. Gently roll back as far as you can without straining, and then slowly roll back up to a sitting position. If you are very stiff, begin by lying flat on your back; bring only one of your knees to your chest as you inhale and hold while you exhale. Repeat with your other leg. Repeat twice.

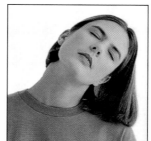

Head rolls
This massages the upper spine. Sit with your back upright and supported. Back, shoulders, and arms should be relaxed. Drop your chin to your chest and slowly rotate your head, first in a clockwise direction, then counterclockwise. Repeat twice.

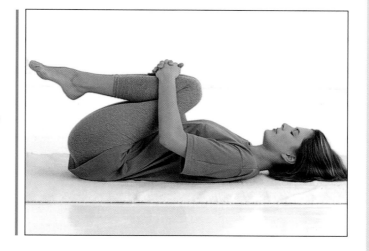

Forward bend
This exercise promotes flexibility of the spine. Sit straight, inhale, and bring both arms above your head. Pause, exhale, and slowly lower your arms toward your toes, gently bending forward from the hips without straining. Repeat twice.

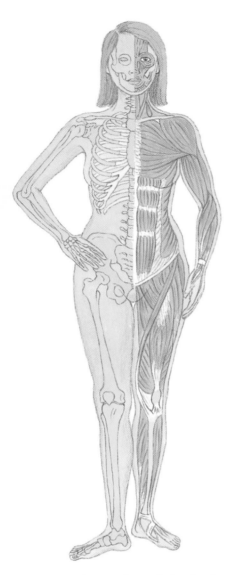

Bones and muscles

The bones and muscles of the body are the key components that enable us to move. Our bones provide us with a rigid internal framework that acts as scaffolding for the body; without our bones we would look something like jellyfish. Bones also play an important role in protecting the vulnerable organs of the body. For example, the skull encloses the brain and the rib cage protects the delicate tissues of the heart and lungs.

For its strength, bone is astonishingly light. If the skeleton were built to the same strength but made of steel, it would weigh about five times as much. Part of this strength comes from the way that bones are constructed. The outsides—especially at load-bearing areas such as the joints—are made of dense, hard bone, while the inside is a lacy honeycomb of bone that combines sufficient structural strength with supreme lightness.

Bone is living tissue made of protein and collagen, a tough, strong, rubbery substance made rigid by calcium and phosphorus salts. Just like the other tissues of the body, these living bones need nourishment and so they are laced with a network of blood vessels that feed them oxygen and nutrients.

Bone is also capable of changing. For instance, if we exercise a lot, the bones become stronger at the places where they are put under stress. If we break a bone it will repair itself by making new bone just as strong, if not stronger, than the surrounding bone. There is, in fact, a constant process of dissolving and reconstructing of bone going on in our bodies, with the essential nutrients, including minerals, being moved from site to site by our blood. This process slows down as we become older, but can be combated by continued exercise.

Bones and muscles of the body

Most adults have 206 bones and these make up about 15 percent of our total weight. Bones range in length from the tiny stapes, or stirrup, in the inner ear, which is about the size of a rice grain, to the thigh bone, or femur, which is over one-quarter the height of an adult.

There are approximately 640 muscles involved in making us move. In the average man muscles make up nearly half of body weight and in the average woman slightly more than one-third. The biggest muscle in both men and women is the gluteus maximus of the buttocks.

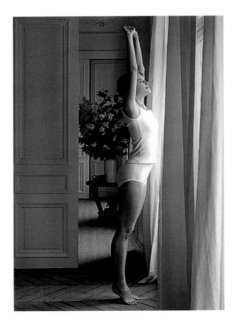

Stretching and toning

Stretching and toning exercises keep the muscles flexible and help joint mobility, making it easier to maintain a proper, relaxed posture. Bones and muscles, and the tissues that connect them to each other, work together to maintain posture. Strong muscles take the weight-bearing strain off the bones when lifting heavy objects by protecting the joints of the back, knees, and shoulders. Poor posture can lead to problems with the spine, resulting in backache, neck pain, and other joint problems. Firm stomach muscles will help to support the spine, and exercising, stretching, and toning the whole body will make good posture much easier to maintain.

The muscles

The muscles that allow us to move about are the voluntary muscles, so called because they are under our voluntary control. They are connected to the bones of the skeleton; nerves send them signals to instruct them to move.

Muscles work by getting shorter. When a signal is sent from the brain along a nerve to a muscle, it contracts. This contraction uses up energy that is supplied by glucose, or sugar. In the process of a complex chemical reaction, oxygen is needed to release the energy stored in the sugar. This is why the increased energy used in our muscles when we exercise vigorously makes us breathe harder to get more oxygen to the muscles via the lungs and blood.

Generally, the larger a muscle is, the more power it has to work. But unless you need big muscles for repeated strenuous work, or want them for cosmetic reasons, healthy muscles are simply those that are toned up by regular exercise.

Dietary tips for muscles

Muscles need protein for growth and carbohydrates for energy. But this does not mean that a person wishing to have healthy muscles needs to go on a high-protein diet. Neither does it mean that someone who does not exercise much will have stronger muscles after eating a lot of starchy foods. In fact, a balanced diet will give your muscles all that they need. However, if you get a great deal of exercise regularly, you will need to eat extra carbohydrates—especially complex carbohydrates—to give you the extra energy required.

Foods to include in your diet
● High carbohydrate foods, such as pasta, rice, bread, and potatoes.
● Fresh fruits and vegetables, including bananas, a good quick source of energy.

Foods to avoid in your diet
● Alcohol—it can harm the muscles.
● Sugar-sweetened snacks.
● Fatty foods, especially animal fat.

Osteoporosis

The word "osteoporosis" means "porous bones" and the problem occurs when more bone tissue is lost than is replaced. Osteoporosis is a common medical condition linked to the aging process, when the level of bone density begins to fall and bone loss accelerates. The bones get thinner, making them more fragile and thus vulnerable to injury. Osteoporosis affects posture and mobility and makes the bones more likely to fracture.

Bone mass is progressively lost from the age of 30 onward, particularly in women—almost one in three women will suffer from osteoporosis. Women suffer a further increased loss of bone during menopause, when they are no longer producing the hormones that help maintain the balance of bone loss with new bone formation. However, this loss can be considerably made up by regular exercise, particularly weight-bearing exercises, and a calcium-rich diet with adequate amounts of magnesium.

How to avoid osteoporosis

Osteoporosis can be avoided or alleviated; regular exercise and a diet rich in calcium and adequate amounts of magnesium, are the keys to controlling it.

● Eat a regular, varied, and fresh diet throughout your life. Younger women should be sure they always get enough calcium, found in dairy products and edible fish bones such as those in sardines.
● Women over the age of 30 and women who have reached menopause should consider taking calcium supplements to help combat potential losses of calcium.
● Exercise regularly to help build up bone density. Weight-bearing exercises build strong bones.
● Minimize stress in your life.
● Avoid refined processed foods, coffee, tea, carbonated beverages, sugar, salt, and alcohol.
● Do not diet excessively or allow yourself to become too thin. Thin women are much more likely to develop osteoporosis than heavy women.

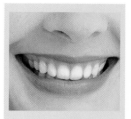

Tips for healthy teeth

The permanent adult teeth are the last natural ones we get. They need looking after to prevent decay and disease and, worst of all, extraction. There are some common-sense rules for dental health that should be followed:

● Brush teeth with a fluoride toothpaste at least twice a day.

● Floss after brushing to remove food and plaque between the teeth.

● Avoid sugar-sweetened snacks and carbonated beverages—many of these contain high amounts of sugar.

● Visit your dentist for a checkup and cleaning twice a year.

● Teeth need calcium, so make sure you get enough in your diet.

The Immune System

Every minute of every day we come into contact with countless disease-causing organisms. They are in the air we breathe, the food we eat, and the liquid we drink. Protecting us from this potentially deadly microscopic onslaught is an extraordinary, multilayered defense system called the immune system. Without a healthy immune system we would not survive for very long.

The immune system depends on white blood cells to function. These cells organize and mount our resistance to infection and therefore play a vital role in keeping us fit and well. White blood cells are made in the spleen, tonsils, adenoids, and bone marrow as well as in the glands of the lymphatic system.

The lymphatic system is a key component of the immune system. Part of its role is to collect and drain excess fluids from the spaces between the body's cells. During the process it filters out bacteria, viruses, and other foreign material. This happens at the lymph nodes—glands that act as filters, sorting out any disease-causing material. The lymph glands are also factories, busy producing our natural weapon against disease. Because of their role in fighting infection, the lymph glands often swell up as the immune system swings into action, providing one of the first signs of illness. The lymph nodes contain white blood cells that can recognize and destroy bacteria and other unwanted particles or cells.

One type of white cell—the B cell—makes antibodies to specific invaders that cling to them, tagging the invader for destruction. Other white cells—T cells—have a complex role in recognizing and destroying specific invaders or foreign material and in activating other cells, including engulfing cells and so-called natural killer cells, to destroy them.

The readiness and effectiveness of the immune system can change, however. One way this can happen is in response to our state of mind. Research has shown that stress, deep grief, and depression can make us more likely to become ill. Conversely, laughter has been found to boost immune system function. If you are feeling low or cannot manage stress properly, you should not only take practical steps such as reducing your work load, but you should also aim to alter your state of mind. Consider learning positive-thinking techniques and assertiveness training or, for tough cases, counseling or therapy. Research has also shown that when it comes to fighting serious illnesses, such as cancer, those with a positive frame of mind will do better than those who feel that they are beaten, or who feel like giving up the fight.

There are simple things that we can do to look after our lymph system, including eating a balanced diet and exercising regularly, while various natural treatments, such as aromatherapy, can have an excellent effect on reducing stress.

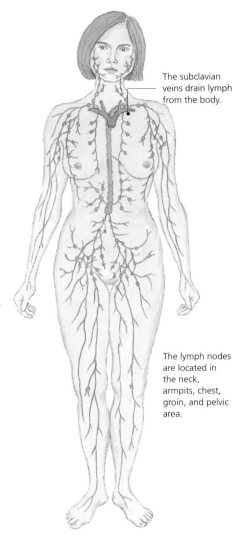

The subclavian veins drain lymph from the body.

The lymph nodes are located in the neck, armpits, chest, groin, and pelvic area.

The lymphatic system

The lymphatic system contains white blood cells that "eat" bacteria and other foreign matter and debris, clearing them from the body. The system drains the body of excess fluid and returns it through the chest to the circulatory system. One-way valves in the lymph vessels ensure lymph flow is in the correct direction. Flow is helped along by muscular movement throughout the body.

Effects of lowered immunity

There are times when the immune system might not function as well as it should. When this happens we are more likely to get sick. For example, we are more prone to catching viral illnesses, such as colds and flu, or developing allergic responses, such as itching and swelling, and more prone to infections such as conjunctivitis. Lowered immunity is, in most people, a temporary state and can be adjusted by rest, relaxation, and eating a well-balanced diet. But for those with AIDS, a disease where the immune system is attacked by the HIV virus, the lowering of immunity is catastrophic and many other so-called opportunistic infections such as viral, bacterial, or fungal infections can occur and prove fatal.

In other cases the immune system can decide to turn on the body and attack it as if it were foreign tissue. These autoimmune diseases include rheumatoid arthritis, Type I diabetes, and systemic lupus erythematosus.

Manual lymph drainage

Manual lymph drainage is an extremely light, repetitive, hands-on massage treatment that moves the skin across and along the lymph pathways to increase the movement of the lymphatic system, throwing its powers of cleaning, regeneration, and healing into high gear.

At the same time, it affects the nervous system by instigating a change from the normal stressed daytime state to the nighttime state we use when we are asleep. This strengthens the immune system and stimulates the lymphatic system to relax and refresh us.

MLD treatment can increase our resistance to colds, infections, and flu and is good for anyone congested by a bad diet, sedentary lifestyle, and exposure to pollutants. Scars after surgery are also greatly improved with treatment. A few of the many other conditions improved by MLD are: rapid aging, slack and lifeless skin, water retention, constipation, stiff muscles and joints, congested ears and sinuses, swollen ankles, legs, and eyes, and premenstrual swelling and discomfort.

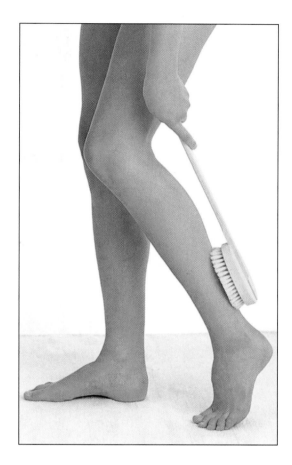

Skin brushing

A quick and simple way to help your lymphatic system is by brushing the skin with a moderately stiff brush, such as one you might use to scrub your back. This can have the effect not only of toning up your skin but also of giving your immunity a boost. It must be done with a dry brush on dry skin and is best done after exercise and before a bath or shower.

Starting at the foot, brush lightly up to the ankle, continuing upward toward the top of your leg. Then do the other foot and leg. Now move on to the arms. Start brushing from the fingers and continue up to the shoulder, covering the whole arm. Use the brush to move down the back. Finally, brush down the front of your body, brushing downward from the shoulders to the level of your hips.

Immune system tips

By keeping your immune system in good shape you'll remain healthier. To do this you should:

• Deal with stress as soon as it comes along. A bad reaction to stress can lower the activity of your immune system.

• Exercise to boost the activity of the immune system.

• Eat a well-balanced diet with plenty of fruits and vegetables.

• If your immune system is depressed take antioxidant vitamins and multivitamins with minerals, especially those containing zinc.

• Avoid excessive exercise since this can actually depress the action of the immune system.

Digestion

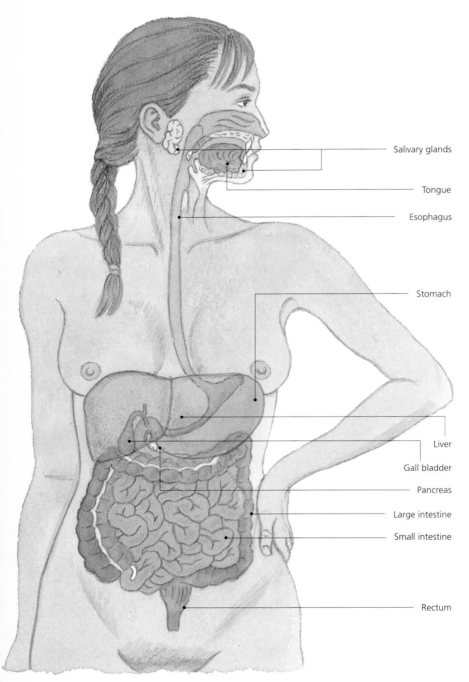

The nourishment we need for our body and mind comes, naturally enough, from the food and drink we consume. We need food for energy and to provide us with essential components to build, repair, and maintain the body. But while we can survive on almost any foodstuffs, eating a nutritionally balanced diet will improve our health and well-being.

Before nutrients can be used by the body they have to be broken down into small units by the digestive system and then absorbed. Chewing food stimulates the production of saliva, which not only makes it easier to swallow food but also contains an enzyme that begins to digest food. Once food is chewed, we swallow. It moves into the throat and then down the esophagus and into the stomach, where it is temporarily stored and further digested. The stomach secretes hydrochloric acid, which kills bacteria, helps dissolve food, and mixes with other chemicals to form a digestive enzyme, pepsin, that starts the breakdown of proteins. The next stop is the duodenum, the first part of the small intestine. Here, partially digested food mixes with digestive juices from the gall bladder and the pancreas. The protein pieces are further broken down to their amino-acid building blocks, while starches and some sugars are broken down by enzymes into simpler sugar units such as glucose. With the food now broken down to its smallest components, absorption can take place. Some absorption takes place in the duodenum but most happens in the rest of the small intestine. The last phase of the process occurs in the large intestine. The remainder of the food solution loses much of its water content here, sheds some more nutrients, and feeds the healthy bacteria living in the intestine. By the time what we have eaten is ready to be excreted, almost all its goodness has been extracted and used by the body.

Labels on illustration: Salivary glands, Tongue, Esophagus, Stomach, Liver, Gall bladder, Pancreas, Large intestine, Small intestine, Rectum

The digestive process
The digestive tract processes food and drink, absorbs nutrients, and gets rid of wastes from the food we eat. Only a small percentage of nutrients are unable to be processed and used by the body from the food as it makes its way through the digestive system.

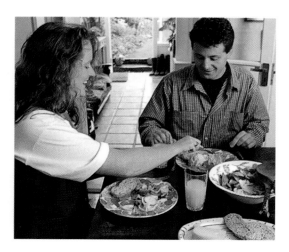

Food digestion times

Different types of food take different amounts of time to digest. While the average digestion time for food is three to four hours, it takes less than two hours for the stomach to process fruits and vegetables. However, proteins, starches, and fats take considerably longer and fatty red meat may spend five to six hours in the stomach before being ready to move on. The total time food spends in the small intestine is about eight hours, and in the large intestine about 12 hours. Food is propelled along at its fastest in the small intestine.

The liver and kidneys

The liver plays an important role in the digestive system and is one of the most important organs of the body. It not only regulates the numerous chemicals in the bloodstream but also acts as a factory, making many of the body's essential chemicals. The liver also deals with toxins, either breaking them down or altering them so they become harmless or can be excreted. The liver acts as a store for glucose, the vital energy supplier, releasing it when needed and storing it when not.

The liver also deals with the levels of amino acids (protein building blocks). If there are too many it alters them chemically into glucose, proteins, other amino acids, or makes them into urea, a waste product that is then filtered from the blood and excreted by the urinary system. Excessive alcohol consumption can impair the functioning of the liver, leading to cirrhosis.

The other main excretion system has the kidneys at its core. To a large extent the two kidneys control the body's fluid balance. They also act as the main organs of liquid-waste disposal. The blood constantly passes through the kidneys and is filtered of urea and other waste chemicals. These, along with any excess water, are passed by a system of tubes to the bladder prior to excretion. The kidneys not only get rid

of excess water but conserve water if the blood is too concentrated. For example, if you drink an excess of fluids the kidneys will get rid of the excess. Similarly, if you have been sweating heavily on a hot day and have not drunk enough water to replace the loss, the kidneys will not excrete much water but will reabsorb it into the body again.

How to avoid irritable bowel syndrome

Irritable bowel syndrome is one of the most common disorders of the intestine. The symptoms can include both constipation and diarrhea, and irregularity. These symptoms usually occur in the absence of other diseases. Symptoms can come and go but may be a lifelong problem. In the absence of other symptoms, it is unlikely to lead to complications but can be distressing. Although the cause is not yet fully understood, you can help reduce its effects by:

● Learning relaxation methods, such as yoga and meditation, to combat stress.
● Eating a high-fiber diet with plenty of bran.
● Regular exercise, which means at least three times a week.
● Drinking a juiced combination of carrot, apple, and celery to help alleviate the symptoms caused by irritable bowel syndrome.

Tips for a healthy digestive system

If you are vulnerable to any foods known to irritate the digestive system, don't eat them. These foods include:

● Fatty meat, fried foods, and saturated fats, such as butter and lard.
● White flour products.
● Strong spices.
● Tea, coffee, alcohol, and carbonated beverages.
● Sugar.
● Salt.
● Wheat gluten (bread).
● Junk food.

● Don't overeat. This exhausts the body by putting too much strain on the digestive system.

● Eat a varied diet high in fresh raw fruits, vegetables, and grains.

● Quit smoking. It may be a major influence in some digestive tract cancers.

● See your doctor, naturopath, or nutritionist if you have any chronic condition that is linked to your digestive system.

Skin and Hair

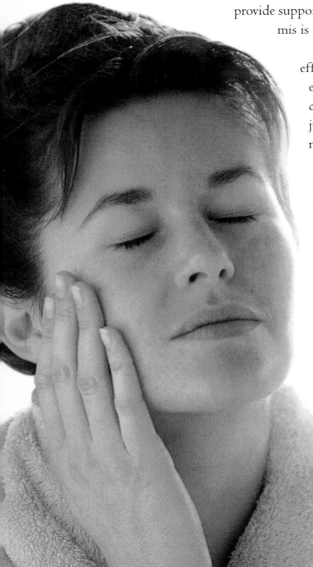

To help conserve the skin's natural moisture it is essential to apply moisturizer after washing. Daily lubrication will help protect the skin against bad weather, environmental hazards, and deterioration of the skin's layers, keeping it soft and smooth. Whatever your skin type, it is worth using a moisturizer containing sunblock to shield the skin from the damaging rays of the sun.

The largest organ of our body is on the outside—it is our skin. It acts as a protective, waterproof, flexible, sensitive, self-repairing barrier between the outside world and all the other organs of our body. Skin regulates our temperature by sweating and keeps out unwanted foreign agents that might cause infection. Our skin also brings us great enjoyment and sensual pleasures through the tiny sense organs involved in the power of touch. It also warns us of danger through pain.

Skin is made up of three layers. The outer, visible layer (epidermis) is made of dead cells. Beneath the epidermis is an inner living layer (dermis). The dead cells are tough and provide a protective layer. They continuously flake off, being replaced by new cells from below. If we injure this top layer of skin it will heal without leaving a scar. The inner layer contains blood vessels, sweat glands, nerves, and layers of collagen that provide support, keeping the skin firm and supple. Below the dermis is a layer of protective subcutaneous fat.

Over time, our skin inevitably suffers some of the effects of stress, harsh weather, too much sun, and environmental pollution. It can also be affected by cigarette smoke, too much alcohol, sweets and other junk food, lack of exercise, and not enough sleep. It might also be missing the care it needs.

But if, as adults, we had a completely blemish-free skin, it would mean that we had not really lived our lives, for the skin and its wrinkles speak of life, experience, and character. Nevertheless, we all aspire to youthful-looking and healthy skin, and fortunately there are some simple rules we can follow to reduce wear and tear. Our skin constantly accumulates dirt, grime, old make-up, sweat, dead cells, and oil. Although this accumulation is not easily seen by the naked eye it will lead to a bacteria build-up and possible skin problems. A clean skin is less likely to suffer from problems, so make skin cleansing and moisturizing a regular part of your morning and evening health rituals. Take care of your skin by protecting it from the sun, harsh winter winds, and the chemicals and detergents found in some soaps.

Tips for healthy skin

- Do not smoke.

- If you have sensitive skin use hypoallergenic skin-care products, especially soaps.

- Always apply a moisturizer after washing your face.

- A balanced diet, rich in fresh fruits and vegetables, will provide all the nutrients you need for healthy skin. Deficiencies of A, B C, and E vitamins may cause skin problems.

- Watch out for any changes in the skin, such as the growth or itching of a mole. Look out for new moles and any changes to the texture of the skin. If these occur consult your doctor.

- Stay out of the hot sun, or if you have to go out, use a high-factor sunblock to prevent skin cancer and premature aging. If you want a deep tan color, use an "indoor tanning" lotion rather than the sun's harmful rays.

Healthy hair

Growing from the subcutaneous layer below the skin of the body is hair. Hair on the head is most obvious and an adult has about 120,000 hairs growing from the scalp, but hair grows on every part of the body except for the palms, soles of the feet, lips, and tip of the penis.

Contrary to what many people think, our hair is not alive—at least not the part of the hair we can see. It is made of a protein called keratin, which is rooted in a tube-shaped depression called the follicle. At the bottom of the follicle is the root where the keratin shaft of a hair is produced. If the root is damaged, the hair may cease to grow. While hair normally grows almost half an inch a month, every so often it goes into a dormant phase. During this time we shed our hair more frequently and you will probably notice when you wash your hair or brush it that more hairs are left behind in the basin or on your hairbrush. However, once the dormant phase is over, hair production begins again. Temporary hair loss can occur through illness, hormonal changes after childbirth, using the contraceptive pill, or by having chemotherapy treatment for cancer. Also, during and after menopause hair tends to become thinner and remains that way.

Hair color is determined by the amount of melanin (a pigment produced at the base of the hair follicle) present in the hair shaft. Various combinations of red-yellow and black-brown melanin determine whether we are redheads, blonds, or brunettes. However, as we grow older, less pigment is deposited in the hair shaft and so gray hairs appear. The age at which we begin to turn gray is very much determined by heredity—some people begin going gray in their early twenties.

Hair analysis

Some practitioners claim to be able to detect dietary deficiencies and other illnesses by using hair analysis. A cutting of hair is treated so that it dissolves and is broken down into its component chemicals, the various proteins that make up the hair. The relative amounts of these proteins are thought to give clues as to any deficiencies in the diet. Other substances found in the hair can reveal whether or not there are toxins in the blood. Following hair analysis, a change in diet or lifestyle may be recommended.

To promote healthy, glowing hair, massage your scalp whenever you wash your hair. This encourages blood to flow to the roots where the hair grows. Using your usual shampoo, gently work from the base of your neck toward the crown of your head, using your fingertips and moving in small circles. Work back down, again using small circles, toward your ears. Follow this by massaging the front of the head. When finished, rinse out the shampoo as usual.

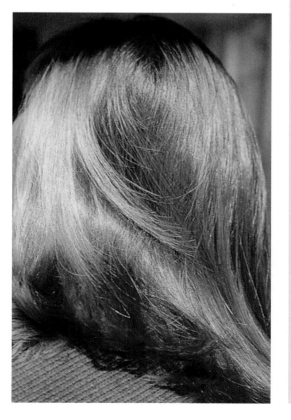

- Wash with the gentlest shampoo suitable for your hair.

- Use a conditioner. These coat the hair with substances that make it bulkier, shinier, and more easy to manage.

- Use hairdryers with care. Use a cool setting and hold the dryer at least six inches away. Avoid using heated rollers and curling irons too much as they can damage the hair ends.

- Keep hair out of the sun and sea if possible or wash and condition immediately afterward.

- Dieting can make hair very dry and straw-like. Make sure you are getting all the vitamins and minerals you need for a balanced diet.

- Perms, dyes, and other treatments are best left to the professionals.

- Regularly cutting hair won't make it grow faster, but it will make the ends stronger and thicker.

The Reproductive Organs

Man's urge to reproduce is very strong: At each male ejaculation approximately 500 million sperm are released, when only one is required to fertilize the female egg. Sperm are produced in the man's testes (testicles) and each one takes about 60 days to form. In contrast, a woman is born with all her eggs in storage in the ovaries and usually only one is released in each menstrual cycle. For fertilization to take place, the sperm, after entering the vagina, must swim past the cervix, through the uterus, and up the fallopian tube at just the right time to meet the egg, which is wafted down the tube by tiny, hairlike fibers. Thus sexual intercourse around the time of ovulation has the best chance of resulting in pregnancy.

According to some researchers (but by no means all) the amount of sperm generated by normal men has fallen by half in the last 50 years. This might be due to so-called environmental estrogens—substances from certain pesticides, industrial chemicals, and some plastics—that are thought to damage the growing fetus, including cells involved in sperm production. As yet no one knows how this may affect human fertility in the future.

Staying well

An overall feeling of well-being depends on many factors. One of the most important of these is your sexual health, which contributes a great deal to your self-image and happiness. The reproductive organs, like other parts of the body, function best if your general health is good, so a balanced diet, exercise, and sufficient rest and sleep all play a part in maintaining your sexual well-being.

Be alert to potential health problems and deal promptly with any discomfort or itching. There are simple, effective treatments available—both conventional and alternative—to relieve minor problems such as thrush and cystitis. For more serious conditions, such as sexually transmitted diseases, you need expert treatment as quickly as possible, not only to avoid passing them on to others but also to ensure that your own fertility is not impaired.

Women should have a Pap smear regularly (once a year for most women) and perform a breast self-examination, as explained at right, each month. Men should seek a checkup at the first sign of urinary-tract or prostate trouble, such as difficulty or pain on urination. They should also seek help if suffering from impotence. In most cases the cause is psychological rather than physical; both can usually be treated successfully.

Breast examination

Regular self-examination of the breasts enables you to detect any changes in them that might need to be investigated by a doctor. While most changes discovered are harmless, any changes that you do detect should be investigated at once. Examine your breasts every month, just after the end of your period.

Strip to the waist and stand in front of a mirror. Look for any noticeable changes in size and whether one breast has recently become lower than the other one. Look at the skin of the breasts for any puckering, dimpling, rashes, or changes in texture. Lift each breast and examine it underneath. Raise your hands above your head and watch for any swelling or skin puckering on either the upper breast or around the armpit. Examine each nipple, looking for discharges or any rashes or skin changes.

Next, lie down with your head and shoulders supported by a pillow and your left hand under your head. Examine your left breast with the flat of your right hand. Slide your hand above and below the nipple, from the armpit to the center of the body, gently pressing to feel for lumps.

Pass your hand from the base of the breast, across the nipple, and upward to the armpit. Slide your hand across your breast and over the nipple. Finally, feel in your armpit and the top of your collarbone. Once completed, repeat the same process for the right breast.

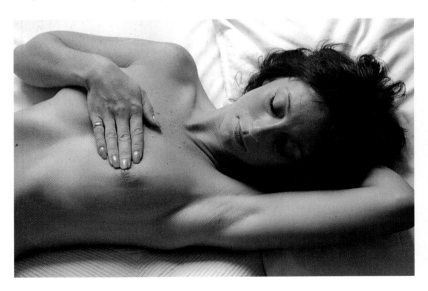

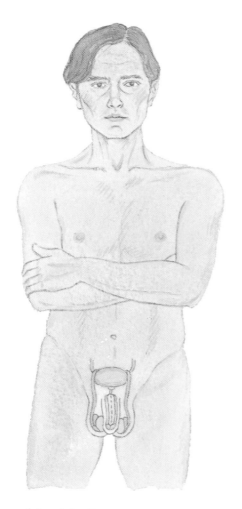

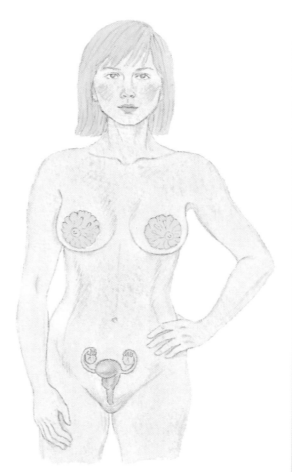

Sexual health for men

• Reduce alcohol intake to improve potency and eat a healthy, well-balanced diet containing plenty of fresh fruits and vegetables.
• Do not smoke.
• Eat a low-fat diet. Fat can reduce the amount of essential male hormones in the blood.
• Exercise regularly as this will increase overall energy levels.
• Avoid wearing tight trousers and underwear. This might help improve sperm levels by keeping the testes cool.
• If you are uncircumcised wash the penis with extra care, especially the tip and foreskin.
• Examine your testicles when the scrotum is relaxed–in the bath, perhaps–looking for any unusual lumps or a change in texture. If you find any, seek medical advice at once.
• There is evidence that free radical oxidants from pollution can damage sperm quality and production. Take a vitamin E supplement and at least 250 mg of vitamin C a day to help combat the effects.

Sexual health for women

• Wash the vaginal area every day, especially if you have an active sex life.
• Don't use vaginal deodorants; they can irritate the skin and cause infections.
• Wear cotton underwear and avoid wearing pantyhose to allow ventilation of the vaginal area.
• Wear a sports bra if you do vigorous physical exercise.
• Have prompt treatment for any sexually transmitted disease. If untreated they can cause infertility.
• Premenstrual syndrome sufferers might find that oil of evening primrose and supplements of vitamin E, vitamin A, and the B-complex vitamins help relieve symptoms.
• If you have heavy periods consult your doctor about taking iron supplements to prevent anemia.
• There is evidence that free radical oxidants caused by pollution can increase the risk of miscarriage. Take 250 mg supplements of vitamin C to combat this.
• Acupuncture may help boost fertility by unblocking energy channels.

Sexual health tips

Sexually transmitted diseases (STDs) such as chlamydia and gonorrhea can impair fertility, particularly among women. If you suspect that disease is present you should seek treatment promptly.

• Always use a condom if you are not 100% sure of your partner's sexual history. STDs can be contracted through unprotected vaginal, oral, or anal sex.

• Women should look out for any itching, discharge, or unpleasant smell in the vaginal area and have it investigated.

• Men should watch for any swelling or soreness at the tip of the penis or any discharge that looks like yellow pus. If present, they should see a doctor for treatment.

• Genital herpes is now a relatively common STD. Sufferers might find relief by taking either a salt bath or an essential-oils bath containing eucalyptus, thyme, and geranium.

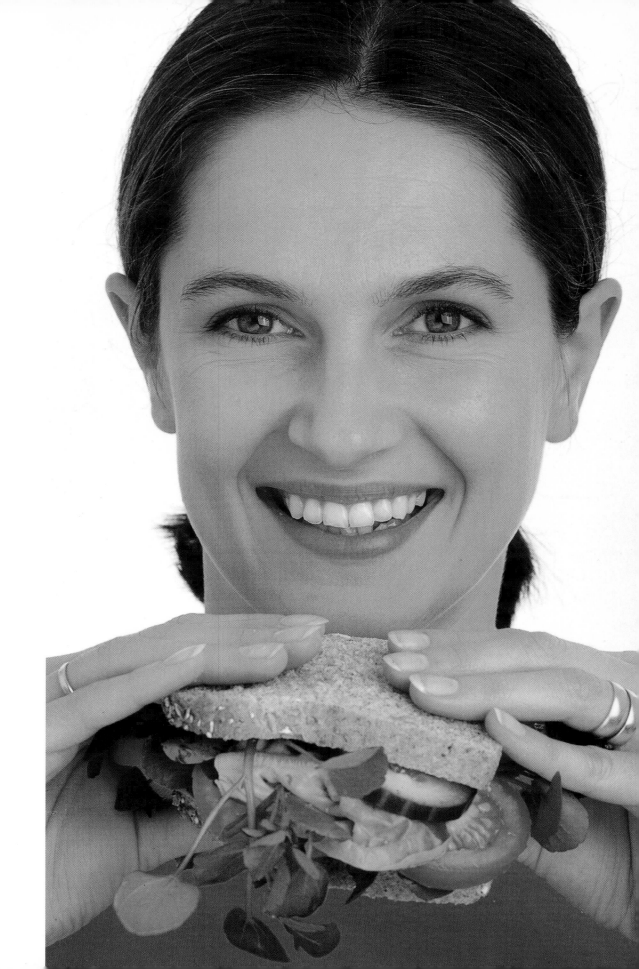

2
Eating Well

The truth is often very simple: If you eat a healthy, balanced diet you can expect to maintain a level of good health. But if you eat too much refined, processed, or junk food and drink too much alcohol you can expect a catalogue of increasing health problems. It is very much to your advantage to consider your personal power in this matter. In most cases you are the keeper of the key that unlocks your ability to keep well and maintain optimum health throughout your life.

There are many ways to eat well. We are lucky that our choice of foods is so varied, but it is our responsibility to create a climate of health within our bodies that will keep us well and prevent chronic health problems. This chapter looks at some of the different ways you can eat well to keep well.

Body Image

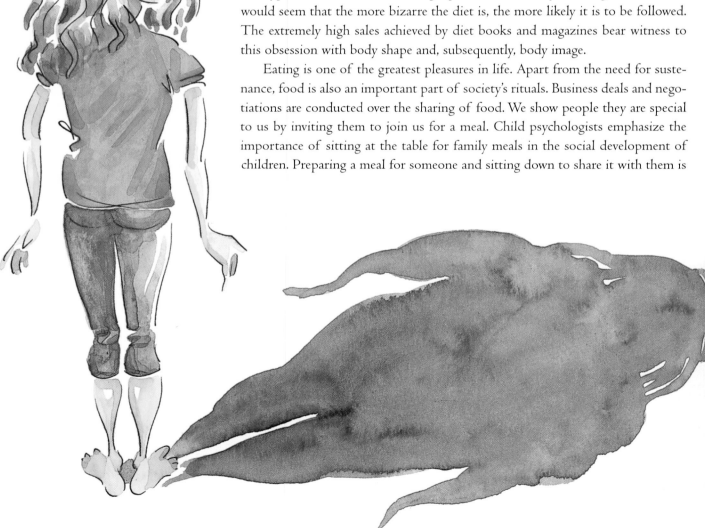

Pressure on women to conform to stereotypes unfortunately means that many become unreasonably dissatisfied with the way they look. This, in turn, adversely affects self-image and promotes feelings of low self-esteem.

So much of our self-image derives from the way we look, rather than from what we are and what we do. This superficial attitude is indoctrinated into us from our early teens onward and endorsed by advertisements from the huge diet-program and cosmetics industries, which must foster anxieties about appearance to sell their products. Our inability to mold our bodies into perfect shapes leads to a sense of low self-worth—a direct result of conditioning absorbed from one another and from the media. Generally, the media promote an impossible image of bodily perfection that, despite our physical or genetic inheritance, we vainly try to emulate. The rising trend toward undergoing cosmetic surgery is the latest manifestation of the desire to conform to stereotypical images of beauty.

The quest to be thin leads some people to follow fad diets, which are based not on nutritional needs but on quack theories—for example, living on one particular type of fruit for a week, eating a potato diet, or only drinking milkshakes. It would seem that the more bizarre the diet is, the more likely it is to be followed. The extremely high sales achieved by diet books and magazines bear witness to this obsession with body shape and, subsequently, body image.

Eating is one of the greatest pleasures in life. Apart from the need for sustenance, food is also an important part of society's rituals. Business deals and negotiations are conducted over the sharing of food. We show people they are special to us by inviting them to join us for a meal. Child psychologists emphasize the importance of sitting at the table for family meals in the social development of children. Preparing a meal for someone and sitting down to share it with them is an act of caring; it feeds us on more than the physical level. So if food is such a pleasure and so important, why does it cause so much anxiety and guilt, particularly among women?

We have a strong relationship with food. Sometimes it is good, sometimes it is bad. We expect food to negotiate with us—for example, if we deny ourselves food we hope to get a model-like figure, which in turn will allow us to find the ideal partner. This is a pretty tall order to expect food to achieve. In the most extreme cases food can be used as a weapon: By denying ourselves an adequate amount of food, we can punish ourselves or others.

Eating is one of the most guilt-producing activities we indulge in. We feel guilty because we eat too much of the wrong foods. A chocolate bar is a secret treat, eaten furtively and then regretted. Hours of exercise or fasting can result from the guilt caused by this one tiny indulgence.

All food fads and severe dieting regimens can lead to nutritional disorders. We may shift a lot of fat on a diet, but we also lose in the texture and condition of our hair, skin, and nails, lack energy and vigor, and are more prone to illness. And, of course, strict dieting regimens are inevitably prone to failure. By concentrating so much on food, it begins to take over our lives. That sneakily eaten chocolate bar takes on a significance disproportionate to its true value.

Overcoming an obsession with our body image may not be easy but it starts with beginning to accept ourselves for what we are, a little bit flawed, maybe a little bit overweight, but unique and worthy. However, if our excess weight is gained by eating an unhealthy diet and following an inactive lifestyle then we *can* do something positive about it. We can follow a healthier eating plan; and if our levels of fitness are low, we can begin to exercise. If our self-esteem is low we can actively change our attitude toward ourselves by consciously adopting a more positive approach to ourselves and our lives.

We should be realistic about our goals. Honest diet experts will tell you that although it is possible to follow a low-calorie diet and lose weight, unless you have a nutritionally balanced eating plan and are sensible about how much you can lose *safely*, your health will suffer. If you need to lose weight, count the calories by all means but follow a nutritious diet, replacing the unhealthy calories with vitamin- and mineral-packed, energy-inducing foods. And don't be afraid to allow yourself an occasional treat. Food, like life, should be enjoyed!

Eating disorders

At its most extreme a negative self-image can become so distorted that it threatens life itself. The increase in the incidence of serious eating disorders such as anorexia nervosa and bulimia dramatically demonstrates the problems and the dangers of a distorted and unrealistic body image.

Most eating disorders are of mental, rather than physical, origin. Although the eating disorder may initially have been triggered by illness, stress, or dieting, many sufferers use their disorder as a weapon to punish either themselves or others. So powerful are their feelings of self-loathing for having done or not done something—not been pretty enough, not lost enough weight, not done well enough in their exams, been the cause of parental arguments—that they decide either to punish themselves through not eating or to punish others by not eating: "Look what *you've* done to me."

Sometimes an eating disorder is used as a form of control. Many believe that although they are powerless over events that occur in their lives, they can at least exert control over their bodies.

Severe eating disorders always need medical and psychotherapeutic attention, but treatment can be backed up by many alternative therapies: hypnotherapy to alter the perceived self-image; acupuncture to relieve stress and rebalance the body's energy; naturopathy to reeducate ideas about nutrition; and autosuggestion to promote a positive self-image. All these alternative therapies have a role to play in helping the sufferer gain a positive attitude toward his or her body image.

The Balanced Diet

The key to achieving optimum health, feeling good, and looking great is eating a balanced diet that is rich in vitamins and minerals. In order to work efficiently our bodies require these nutrients on a daily basis. Although we are all different in shape, size, and age, we all need the same basic nutrients—the vitamins, minerals, carbohydrates, fiber, protein, and fats that nourish and energize us.

Generally, we should eat more fresh fruits and vegetables, more whole-grain bread, pasta, grains and cereals, and more lean meat and fish. We should eat less red meat and fatty foods, refined flour and sugar products such as cakes, cookies, and white bread. We should try to avoid junk food, salt, and processed products, which are often high in added salt and preservatives. We should also try to drink fewer caffeine-containing drinks, such as coffee and colas, and sugar-sweetened drinks. Limiting our alcohol intake also helps us maintain alertness and health.

By eating in this way we can promote good health and help prevent illness and degenerative disease. Eating a wide variety of foods from the four main food groups described on these pages will provide us with all we need to maintain a well-balanced diet, improve our health, increase our fitness and energy levels, and promote a greater sense of well-being.

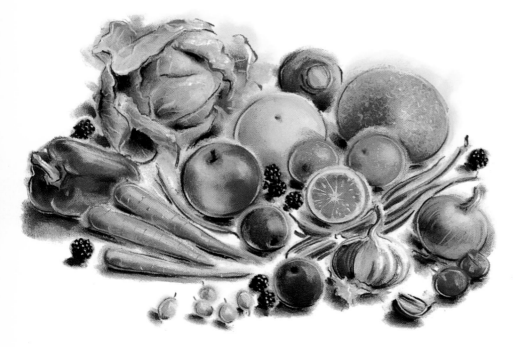

Starchy foods—carbohydrates
These are an excellent source of fiber, B vitamins, and many minerals. They are filling foods that provide us with energy.
- Eat about 5 servings a day.
1 serving = 1 slice of bread, 1 cup of cooked pasta, rice, peas, cooked dried beans or cereal, 1 small potato.
Good carbohydrate sources:
- bread (whole-grain) • cereals (whole grain) • pasta • rice • potatoes • peas and dried beans • seeds.

Fruits and vegetables
Fruits and vegetables have a high vitamin and mineral content. They are the main source of the antioxidant nutrients (vitamins A, C, and E), plus beta carotene and selenium. Many experts believe they help fight illnesses, ranging from the common cold to cancer and heart disease.
- 5 to 6 servings a day.
1 serving = 1 piece of fruit, 1 large portion of vegetables.
Good fruits and vegetables:
- apples • citrus fruits • apricots • pears • pineapple • melon • bananas • grapes • strawberries • avocados • tomatoes • cauliflower • peppers • garlic • carrots and other root vegetables • leafy green vegetables such as broccoli and spinach.

*"Anyone can be as well as desired if given
the right food in the right way."*
WILLIAM HAY, INVENTOR OF THE HAY DIET

Dairy foods

Rich in calcium and phosphorus, dairy foods help to build and maintain strong bones and teeth. They are often high in fat so choose low-fat versions of these foods, such as skim milk and low-fat cheeses.
- Eat 2 to 3 servings a day.
1 serving = 1 pint of milk, 2 to 3 ounces of butter or cheese, 1 small carton of yogurt.
Good dairy food sources:
- butter • cheese • yogurt • milk.

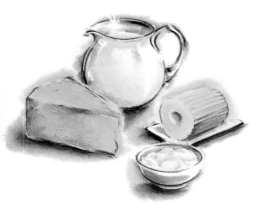

Proteins

Protein helps the body build energy and strength. It is, however, the hardest food for the body to break down and digest, using more energy in the digestion process than any other food. Animal protein is turned into human protein only after it has been digested and turned into amino acids, which the body then uses to create the protein it needs.
- 2 to 3 servings a day.
1 serving = 1 portion of fish, poultry, or lean meat, 3 tablespoons of cooked beans or lentils, 2 eggs (but don't eat more than 4 eggs a week), 2 to 3 ounces of mixed nuts.
Good protein sources:
- fish • poultry
- meat • eggs
- beans • lentils
- soy and tofu
- nuts, such as cashews and almonds.

Food combining

The science of food combining was created early in the 20th century by William Howard Hay, an American doctor who claimed to cure himself and many of his patients of serious illnesses by making dramatic changes in dietary habits. Hay aimed to help people to step out of the way of their own healing by removing "the obstacles in the way of nature's own healing powers."

One of the secrets of his successful food combining regimen is the way fruit is eaten. Foods that are easiest and quickest to digest are alkaline-forming and found in most fruits and vegetables. Foods that are the most difficult to digest are acid-forming foods found in most proteins, starches, and cooked food. As far as possible, fruit should be eaten raw, on an empty stomach, and never with or after other foods. By eating fruit in this way all its goodness and cleansing effects work quickly on the digestive system, detoxifying as they travel.

Another rule is that proteins and starches should not be eaten together because it is too taxing for the digestion. However, they mix very well with vegetables and salad. So, instead of meat and potatoes, have meat and vegetables. The same goes for pasta and rice. These mix well with vegetables but not with each other or with meat. Remember, too, to allow four hours to elapse between meals to allow food to digest properly.

Hay Diet rules

- Starches and sugars should not be eaten with proteins and acid fruits at the same meal.

- Vegetables, salads, and fruits should constitute the major part of our diet.

- Proteins, starches, and fats should be eaten in small quantities.

- Only whole-grain and unprocessed starches should be used.

- An interval of at least four hours should elapse between meals of different character.

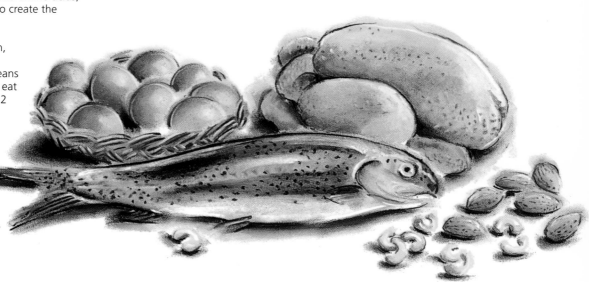

According to the World Health Organization, the everyday diet that is most highly recommended is that eaten by the people of the Mediterranean basin. Traditionally they eat the foods produced in the area: complex carbohydrates in the form of pasta, peas, beans, and rice; plentiful vegetables, particularly the "protective" dark green, yellow, and other brightly colored vegetables, such as broccoli, peppers of all kinds, carrots, pumpkins, and green salads; and similar colored fruits, such as melons, apricots, peaches, nectarines, and oranges. They eat hardly any dairy products (saturated fats) and instead cook with olive oil (monounsaturated fat). Their diet contains only small amounts of protein, mainly in the form of oily fish such as mullet and tuna, which contain omega-3 fatty acids. Complex carbohydrates contain large quantities of fiber, which is known to lower blood cholesterol and reduce the risk of some cancers. The so-called protective vegetables are rich sources of vitamins C, E, and beta carotene, which actively protect against deficiency diseases and heart disease. Omega-3 fatty acids and monounsaturated fats have remarkable powers to lower blood cholesterol and stimulate the action of the pancreas. The Mediterranean diet includes plenty of garlic, whose active ingredient, allicin, appears to be very effective in reducing blood pressure and preventing blood clots.

Protective Mediterranean foods

Mediterranean ingredients are known to be beneficial to health in many ways, particularly their ability to protect against heart disease and various other deficiency conditions detailed below.

Complex carbohydrates
- Grains, e.g., pasta, bulgur, etc.
- Peas, beans, and lentils.
- Root vegetables.
- Nuts and seeds.
- Some fruits and vegetables.
Contain: Fiber.
Benefits: Lower blood cholesterol.
- May protect against some cancers.

Protective fruits and vegetables
- Yellow vegetables, such as peppers, sweet potatoes, carrots, pumpkins.
- Dark green vegetables, such as broccoli, Brussels sprouts, peas, asparagus.
- Leafy vegetables, such as salad greens, spinach, watercress, cabbage.
Contain: Vitamins C and E.
- Beta carotene, which converts to vitamin A.
- Provide good sources of fiber.
Benefits: Free radicals are inactivated.
- Cancers of colon, breast, and lungs are reduced.
- Effects of aging are delayed and reduced.

Fats
- Olive oil.
- Oily fish, such as tuna, mackerel, sardines, mullet, anchovies.
Contain: Monounsaturated fat.
- Omega-3 fatty acids.
Benefits: Lower blood cholesterol.
- Reduce low-density lipoprotein levels.
- Stimulate pancreas to reduce risk of stomach ulcer.

Garlic
Contains: Allicin.
Benefits: Antiseptic/antifungal properties.
- Prevents blood clots. • Destroys free radicals. • Lowers blood pressure.
- Lowers cholesterol.

Mediterranean eating plan

Eating the Mediterranean way is not only healthy, it's also delicious—and the rich, vibrant colors of the food will remind you of lazy, relaxed days in the sun. This one-week eating plan incorporates many typical foods eaten in Mediterranean countries to provide a nutritionally balanced blend of amazing tastes and textures that are low in fat and calories and high in fiber, vitamins, and minerals.

Every day
BREAKFAST

A serving of plain yogurt

A helping of fresh fruit chosen from the following:

   nectarines, peaches, plums, mangoes, oranges, grapefruit, melon, cherries, strawberries, or raspberries

Day one
LUNCH

Pita pockets filled with feta cheese and salad greens

Mozzarella, tomato, and basil salad

DINNER

Mediterranean seafood platter

Banana and strawberry sherbets

Day two
LUNCH

Tapenade dip with a selection of raw vegetables

DINNER

Pasta with fresh pesto sauce

Green salad with oregano-seasoned oil and vinegar dressing

Day three
LUNCH

Seafood salad with fresh citrus dressing

I peach or apricot

DINNER

Mushrooms marinated in garlic sauce

Feta cheese and sliced green bean salad with diced red onion

A slice of Italian olive bread

Strawberries with plain yogurt

Day four
LUNCH

Broad bean and pasta salad with orange and grapefruit dressing

I nectarine, peach, or other piece of yellow or orange fruit

DINNER

Salade niçoise

A chunk of French bread

Chilled melon and strawberries

Day five
LUNCH

Pita pockets of tuna, onions, and diced green pepper

Grapes or strawberries

DINNER

Pasta with broccoli, capers, and Parmesan cheese shavings

Peaches poached in rosé wine

Day six
LUNCH

Crab and melon salad

I apple or other piece of fruit

DINNER

Grilled sardines with broccoli and a tomato and basil salad

Citrus fruit salad and honey

Day seven
LUNCH

Grilled chicken breast with tomato and basil sauce

Couscous

I banana with plain yogurt

DINNER

Shrimp, melon, and avocado salad

Italian bread

Good and Bad Fats

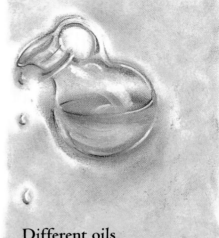

Fats are essential in a healthy diet. They play a vital part in the body's ability to produce energy and to carry and store some vitamins—but we eat far too much of them. The fats we don't use up are turned into fat in our bodies, collecting in all those places we would rather it did not. Apart from weight gain, an excess intake of fats is directly responsible for the high number of heart conditions that exist in our society; excess fat in the blood causes plaque to form on our artery walls, which leads to heart disease.

It is easy to eat too much bad fat, given the Western diet. Generally, we eat far too much fatty red meat and too much sugar and refined foods. Is it just coincidence that the huge rise in the manufacture and consumption of junk food in the last 50 years parallels the increased incidence of illnesses connected to dietary excesses?

Experts in the past have said that it is essential to keep our intake of saturated fatty acids down to avoid the risk of heart disease, and that cooking oils and spreads rich in monounsaturates and polyunsaturates are a healthier choice. However, new research is emerging which shows that not all fats, margarines, and spreads made from vegetable oils are in fact healthier. This is because of the presence of trans fatty acids (often called trans fats), which are monounsaturates and polyunsaturates twisted out of their normal molecular shape by hydrogenation, the chemical process that changes oils to spreads, margarine, shortening or solid fats. These are known as trans-formed fats. Several studies have shown that trans fats act on our cholesterol level in much the same way as saturated fats. They raise the level of LDL cholesterol, the "bad" cholesterol, in the blood and reduce the levels of HDL cholesterol, the "good" cholesterol.

Although there are some trans fats that occur naturally in butter and milk, these do not have the same properties as the trans fats found in artificially hydrogenated oils and do not seem to be as dangerous to our health. More research needs to be done before the experts can reach a conclusion, but the findings of various studies have been serious enough to stimulate many manufacturers to reduce the level of trans fats in their products.

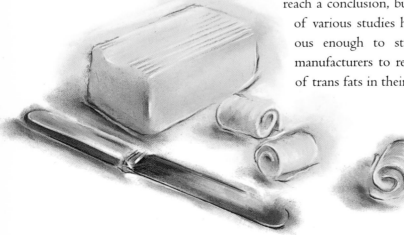

Different oils

Solid oils
These are usually a mix of saturated and unsaturated fats and are generally much lower in saturated fatty acids than butter or lard. However, their total fat content is still on a par with lard and higher than that found in butter.

Olive oil
Olive oil has monounsaturate fat and is the best oil for cooking. Try always to buy olive oil that is labelled "virgin," "extra virgin," or "cold pressed," as these will not have been chemically altered or heat treated, which can convert unsaturates to saturates.

Fish oils
Some fish contain good fats, known as omega-3 oils. These are to be found in fish such as mackerel, sardines and salmon.

Vegetable oils
There are many types of oil of vegetable origin. Apart from olive oil, the best oils to use are rape-seed oil and walnut oil, an expensive but delicious alternative to olive oil in salad dressings.

Types of fat

Given that we need some fat in our diet, which fats should we favor? Diets very low in fat may lack essential fatty acids (EFAs). Tests have shown that people with low blood levels of EFA also had low levels of HDL, the "good" cholesterol that protects against heart disease.

The fatty acids we need come from vegetable oils, such as olive oil and sunflower oil, and omega-3 fatty acids, found in fish oils. All fats are a combination of saturated and unsaturated fats. Saturated fat becomes hard when left at room temperature, while unsaturated fat remains liquid or soft. Saturated fats contain higher amounts of saturates than unsaturated fat and are therefore the type of fat you need to keep in check or reduce in your diet. These fats include butter, hard margarine, lard, coconut oil, palm oil, and animal fat, found in meat.

Unsaturated fats largely fall into two categories: monounsaturated fats, found in olive oil, peanut oil, and rapeseed oil, and polyunsaturated fats, found in oils that come from seeds, nuts, and fish. Polyunsaturates are found in corn oil, soy oil, sunflower and safflower oil, and many margarines.

Fat content found in food

Butter
Made from animal fat and therefore high in saturates, butter is at least 50 percent saturated fatty acids. Low-fat butters have fewer saturates and are therefore preferable.

Lard
Another member of the animal fat family, lard is very high in saturated fat and usually contains around 100 percent saturated fatty acids.

Milk
An 8-ounce serving of whole milk contains 5 g of saturated fat. An easy way to cut down on your daily intake of fat is to substitute 2 percent (3 g sat. fat per 8 oz.), 1 percent or low-fat (1.5 g sat. fat), or skim (0 g sat. fat) milk. Skim milk has a weaker taste than whole and may take some getting used to, but it is the best choice for healthy adults. However, infants and toddlers should have at least 2 percent milk to ensure the development of healthy bones and nervous system.

Yogurt
Depending on the type of yogurt, its saturated fat content can vary widely. Low-fat and fruit yogurts usually contain 1.5 g of saturated fat per 8-ounce serving. Light and plain yogurts generally have 0 g of fat, saturated or unsaturated, per serving. It is best to use plain, unflavored yogurt with active cultures when you are combining yogurt with fresh fruit or with herbs and spices for a salad dressing or dip. Always check the nutritional information on the back of the carton.

Cream
Cream is basically butterfat and is very high in animal, or saturated, fat. You should consider completely eliminating it from your diet. A 2-tbsp. serving of heavy, or whipping, cream contains 6 g of saturated fat. Even table, or light, cream has 3 g sat. fat in a 2-tbsp. serving. Half-and-half is slightly better at 2 g sat. fat per 2-tbsp. serving. Sour cream weighs in at 2.5 g sat. fat per 2-tbsp. serving. There are many varieties of low- and no-fat sour cream that make acceptable substitutes for the high-fat type.

Cheeses
Cheese is generally high in saturated fat but there is often a healthier low-, medium-, or reduced-fat version available. Medium-fat cheeses include edam and goat's cheese as well as some of the soft cheeses such as brie and camembert, feta, and blue-veined cheeses. Low-fat cheeses, such as cottage cheese and ricotta, are the lowest fat. All these cheeses are good alternatives to cream cheese or mayonnaise toppings or dressings that have a high fat content.

White meat
The meat from chicken and turkey–the most common types of white meat–contains less fat than other meats and is a good source of protein. However, there is a much higher amount of fat in the skin of poultry and it should not be eaten on a low- fat diet. Young birds have less fat than older ones.

Red meat
The traditional red meats of beef, lamb, and pork can contain relatively high levels of fat, depending on the cut and on the amount of fat in the meat itself. Typically, roast beef is 40 g of fat per 3½-ounce serving. The fat in meat is mostly saturated fat.

Snacks
Potato chips, cocktail nuts, and dips can be very high in fat. Cakes and cookies can also contain high levels of hydrogenated vegetable oils. Try eating fresh fruit or raw vegetables, such as an apple or carrot sticks, instead.

Healthy fat tips

In an ideal world, no more than one-third of our calories should come from fat—and less than one-third of our fat intake should be from saturated fats. Fats can be good for you because:

• They are a rich source of the fat-soluble vitamins A, D, E, and K.

• They play an important part in making estrogen in women.

• They provide the body with an important source of energy and heat, measured in calories, which burn off during activity.

• They protect and cushion our vital organs and insulate against heat loss. Body fat is important in cold climates but we need less in warm climates.

• They contain linoleic acids that help our bodies make other polyunsaturated fatty acids, which help us metabolize cholesterol.

The Vegetarian Debate

Ever-increasing numbers of people are questioning the wisdom of a meat-based diet and converting to a vegetarian or partly vegetarian diet. There are good health reasons for considering reducing or eliminating our meat intake. Red meat has been linked to the increase in heart disease, cancer, diabetes, gallstones, arthritis, and many other conditions in Westerners who eat meat-rich diets, compared with people of other cultures who eat predominantly grain- or fish-based diets. Eating fruits, vegetables, beans, and peas provides the body with abundant vitamins, minerals, protein, carbohydrates, and very little fat.

Many modern nutritionists and anthropologists believe fruit is the most important food we eat and that it is the one food to which the human species is biologically adapted. Our human ancestors were not predominantly meat eaters, or even eaters of seeds, shoots, leaves, or grasses, but subsisted chiefly on a diet of fruit. Fruit is easy to digest and has a cleansing as well as a nourishing effect on the body because of its high water content, which helps us to "spring clean" our internal organs and systems.

Delicious vegetables and fruit, in conjunction with a balanced diet (page 34), will provide all the nutrients we need for healthy living. Fresh fruits and vegetables also provide fiber, essential for an effective and efficient digestive system. Being able to choose from the abundance of fruits and vegetables available throughout the year means we can never get bored with our menus. Choose and eat only fresh fruits and vegetables, avoiding any that are wrinkled, blemished, or limp. Eat them raw or just lightly cooked so you can benefit as much as possible from their nutrients.

Experts all over the world recommend we follow a diet high in fruits and vegetables, high in fiber and carbohydrates, and low in fat—in fact the type of diet vegetarians eat.

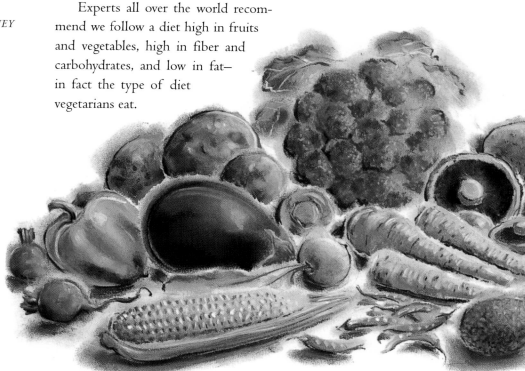

Peas, beans, and lentils

Peas, beans, and lentils contain valuable amounts of protein (vital for the growth and repair of the body and also a valuable source of energy), carbohydrate (the chief source of energy for all body functions), vitamins, minerals, and fiber. In a strict vegetarian diet protein cannot be obtained from the usual sources, such as meat and fish, but has to be obtained from nuts, peas, beans, and foods such as cereals and grains.

When cooked, peas, beans, and lentils have approximately a quarter of the protein content of cheese. They will last for up to a year without losing any of their nutritional value. If bought loose, pick them over to remove any grit or stones. Most dried beans should be soaked before cooking to allow them to soften and regain their original shape and size. They should be washed several times in cold water to remove any dust and then thoroughly boiled to remove the toxins some beans contain. They are also available, cleaned and boiled, in cans. They do not take long to heat through and there is no danger of their having any toxins.

Good beans and peas to try:
- aduki beans • butter beans • brown kidney beans
- red kidney beans • black or white kidney beans
- black-eyed peas • baby lima beans • mung beans
- pinto beans • chickpeas • green lentils • split red lentils • brown lentils.

Nuts and seeds

Nuts and seeds contain protein, fiber, vitamins, particularly B, E, and folic acid, and minerals such as potassium, calcium, magnesium, iron, and zinc. The energy in nuts and seeds is in the form of fat so they should be eaten in small quantities. They should be bought fresh and in small quantities as they dry out when they get old. Store them in airtight containers in a cool, dry place to preserve the oil content.

Good nuts and seeds to try:
- hazelnuts • cashews • almonds • brazil nuts
- pecans • pistachios • walnuts • sesame seeds
- poppy seeds • sunflower seeds.

Grains and cereals

All grains and cereals come from grasses. They are high in fiber and good sources of carbohydrates, protein, and some vitamins and minerals. When eaten in combination with peas, beans, and lentils, grains and cereals provide a well-balanced protein meal. Try to buy the unprocessed types from health food stores.

Good grains and cereals to try:
- brown rice • wild rice • corn • barley • oats • rye
- buckwheat • wheat (including whole wheat, wheat germ, bulgur, bran, semolina, and couscous).

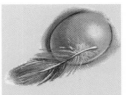

Good egg tips
- Eggs are packed with many valuable food sources—protein, zinc, and B vitamins, as well as other nutrients. But they are also very high in saturated fat, which leads to high cholesterol, so eat no more than four a week.

- If possible, buy free-range eggs. They taste better and the welfare of the egg-producing chickens is given a high priority.

- Because of the high risk of salmonella poisoning, the elderly, pregnant women, children, and those with impaired immune systems should not eat food containing raw eggs, such as homemade mayonnaise and homemade ice cream.

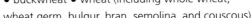

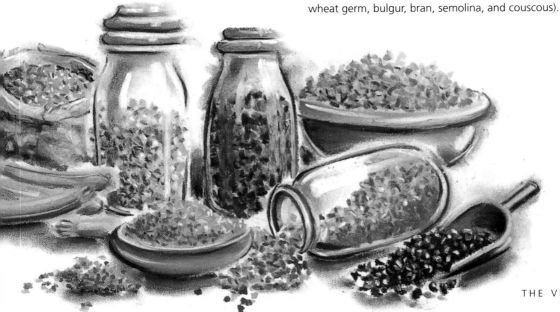

Eat your Greens, Yellows, and Reds...

Growing seeds and sprouts

Seeds and sprouts are highly nutritious–
they rival meat in nutritional value and
tomatoes in vitamin C. Sprouts can be
grown in any climate, take 3 to 5 days to
mature, do not require soil or sunshine, and
may be planted any day of the year. Raw
sprouts have a regenerative effect on our
body and are a storehouse of food energy;
their rich enzyme concentration stimulates
a heightened enzyme activity in our
metabolism, leading to regeneration of
many of our body's processes, particularly
the digestive and circulatory systems.

Good seeds for sprouting
● oat ● buckwheat ● chickpea
● soybean ● alfalfa ● mung bean
● aduki ● wheatgrass ● fenugreek.

How to sprout
Wash the seeds and soak them overnight
in tepid, untreated water. Use two parts
water to one part seeds. Small seeds such
as alfalfa only need to soak for 3 to 6 hours
while larger seeds, such as chickpea and
mung, need soaking for 15 to 20 hours.

Once they are soaked, drain and wash
the seeds again. Place the seeds in a
container in a warm, dark place (60°F to
70°F). While the seeds are sprouting, rinse
them twice a day in tepid water and drain,
putting the container back in its warm,
dark place until ready to eat.

Delicious, colorful fruits and vegetables are packed with easy to absorb nutrients—almost everything the body needs to thrive is contained in them. The body prefers fruits and vegetables because of the ease with which it can digest them, compared with starchy foods and fatty meats. Research has shown that the more fruits and vegetables we eat, the less likely we are to develop cancer or other degenerative diseases.

Green foods contain substances that stimulate the body's immune system and our ability to heal ourselves. Yellow fruits and vegetables are packed with essential nutrients: Carrots have so much beta carotene that you need to eat only one a day to meet your body's requirement for vitamin A, one of the important antioxidants that help keep free radical rogue cells in check. An excellent ally in the battle against high blood pressure and atherosclerosis, carrots also contain daucarine, a substance that stimulates dilation and widening of the arteries. Raw red tomatoes are a rich source of vitamin C, one of the antioxidants, and beta carotene, which is important for balanced cell activity. Fresh tomatoes are also an excellent fiber source and help keep cholesterol levels in check. Recent research from Europe indicates that lycopene, the pigment that makes tomatoes red, may protect the cells from the effects of cigarette smoke and fuel pollution, thereby inhibiting certain cancers from developing. Red peppers are another great source of vitamin C, having the highest content of all fruits and vegetables, and are also packed with beta carotene. Red peppers rank high in the antioxidant war against cancer and heart disease.

When buying fruits and vegetables make sure they are young, fresh, plump, and have a vibrant color. Generally, they should feel heavy for their size. Throw away any that have become blemished, bruised, or wrinkled, since their nutritional content will have become impaired. If vegetables are packed in plastic wrap, remove the covering and then store them in the bottom of the refrigerator or in a cool pantry; there is evidence that some soft plastics contain minute traces of cancer-causing substances that can contaminate the food. Root vegetables like being in the dark, so store them in brown paper bags in the pantry. Fruit should not be stored for longer than two days in the refrigerator. To preserve their goodness, avoid preparing fruits and vegetables too far in advance.

If possible, buy organically grown fruits and vegetables, as pesticide traces are often found in those that are conventionally grown. Pesticides have been linked to various diseases in humans and are thought to have an adverse effect on male fertility. There is also an increasing trend toward irradiating fruits and vegetables to destroy bacteria and prolong shelf life, color, and texture.

...or drink them

Instead of drinking unhealthy teas, carbonated beverages, and alcohol, quench your thirst and increase your liquid intake with a nutritional alternative—fresh fruit and vegetable juice drinks. Your own homemade juice is a totally different taste experience—fresh, clean-tasting, and packed with valuable vitamins and minerals. Your own juices, ideally made using organically grown fruits or vegetables, will be free of preservatives and added sugars, commonly added to commercial juices to preserve their shelf life.

By juicing at home, you can blend together various different fruits and vegetables to make unusual but highly nutritious drinks. These juices are a great way to start the day and will have a powerful, preventive effect on the body. They are ideal for times when the appetite is impaired during bouts of debilitating illnesses such as influenza or the common cold.

Great health juices to try

To juice you need either a centrifuge juicer or citrus press or you can just blend the raw fruits or vegetables in a standard blender, having chopped them up first. All these methods will extract all the goodness of the food into a frothy, delicious, and nutritious treat. Fruits and vegetables without a high water content may need mineral water added.

Celery
High in magnesium and iron, celery helps promote healthy blood cells.

Tomato
High in vitamin C and rich in sodium, calcium, potassium, and magnesium. Helps fight infections and speeds up tissue repair. May help repair the damage caused by fuel pollution and cigarette smoking.

Cranberry
High in vitamin C, with useful amounts of iron, potassium, and vitamin A. Excellent for alleviating the symptoms of cystitis and fatigue.

Apricot
High in beta carotene and iron. Good for the skin and respiratory infections. Some nutritionists believe that apricots help fight cancer.

Papaya
Good for the digestion and said to help blood clotting, papaya juice is also rich in vitamin C.

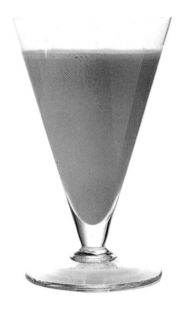

Carrot
Rich in beta carotene, carrot juice increases the level of red blood cells and is said to have a protective action against excess ultraviolet rays.

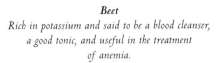

Beet
Rich in potassium and said to be a blood cleanser, a good tonic, and useful in the treatment of anemia.

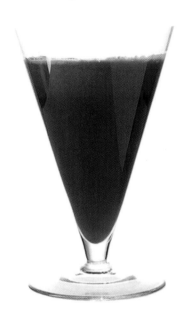

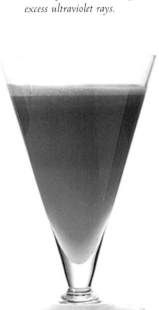

Cucumber
A good diuretic that promotes urine flow. Its high silicon and sulfur content helps hair growth.

Spinach
Spinach is rich in iron, acts as a powerful antioxidant, and is thought to have an important role to play in preventing cancer.

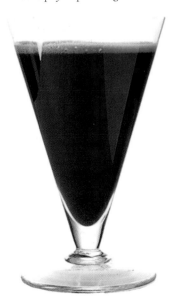

Medicinal and Mood Foods

Mother Nature is infinitely wise in her ways. Many of the ordinary foods we eat possess amazing healing and mood-altering properties. It is not just herbs that have medicinal uses; everyday foods such as cabbage and carrots have healing properties and many plants are used to make medicinal drugs. Plants are used to make strong, usually illegal, mood-altering substances, such as cannabis and cocaine, but they can also be used to help us regulate our own moods by controlling what we eat. Make the foods on this page a regular part of your diet, eating substantial portions to protect your body, prevent serious illness, and achieve a higher level of well-being.

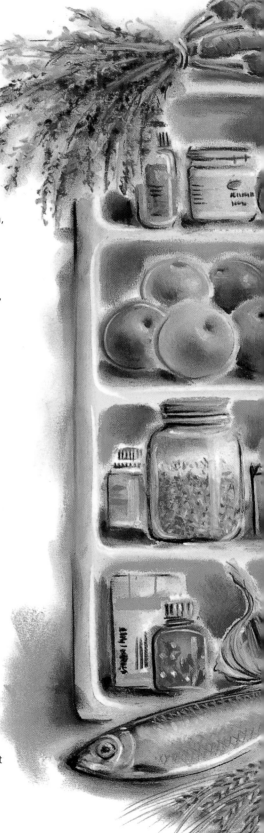

Apples
Some of the acids in apples, such as tartaric acid, help the body cope with too much protein and fatty food and therefore help soothe indigestion.

Avocados
Several studies have confirmed that eating avocados can keep levels of LDL (low-density lipoprotein–the unhealthy part of cholesterol) low.

Broccoli
High in folic acid, broccoli is recommended for those planning to get pregnant and for the first three months of pregnancy; it protects against spina bifida and neural tube defects in the growing child.

Buckwheat
Buckwheat is rich in rutin, which strengthens the walls of the capillaries (the thousands of tiny blood vessels in the body). It is also a good source of fiber and so benefits the digestive system.

Cabbage
Raw cabbage is full of sulfur compounds, which help fight chest infections, and other healing substances that can help cure ulcers in the digestive system. It speeds up estrogen metabolism and is therefore thought to help block breast cancer and suppress the growth of polyps.

Carrots
Packed with beta carotene, carrots help fight infections. They are also said to be effective in reducing strokes in women and reducing the risk of lung cancer in smokers.

Fish and fish oils
These play a vital role in the prevention of heart disease and are said to relieve rheumatoid arthritis, osteoarthritis, asthma, high blood pressure, and psoriasis.

Garlic
This is a powerful healing plant with an excellent reputation for preventing and treating high blood pressure, heart attacks, and strokes. It improves the circulation and helps reduce cholesterol levels and stickiness in the blood–thus reducing the risk of blood clots. It is also a powerful antiseptic when taken internally.

Mustard
The ground seeds of the mustard plant have been used for many centuries to treat colds and chest coughs. Mustard helps break up mucus and so makes a good decongestant and expectorant.

Oats
Oats are rich in nutrients, including calcium, magnesium, and potassium. They help combat high levels of blood cholesterol and also soothe an irritated digestive tract or bowel.

Olive oil
Rich in vitamin E, olive oil is an antioxidant that inhibits the destructive activity of free radicals. Research shows that diets high in extra-virgin olive oil produce a reduction in blood cholesterol levels.

Tomatoes
Very high in vitamin C, tomatoes are also a major source of lycopene, said to act as an anticancer agent. They can be used externally to treat acne.

Yogurt
A calcium-rich source of food, yogurt can help fight osteoporosis and can prevent yeast infections in women.

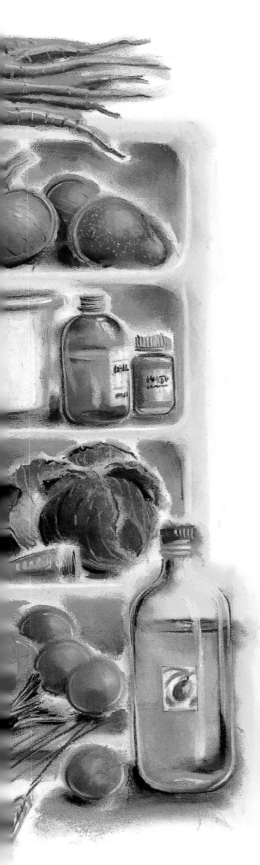

Foods and moods

Because the brain, endocrine, and nervous systems regulate our moods and feelings, and the nutrients we eat feed them, we must assume that what we eat affects our emotions, too. Vitamins and minerals play a major role in our emotional well-being. The brain and nervous system need them all but particularly the B-complex vitamins, which help us utilize the carbohydrates, proteins, and fat we eat. They ensure a continuous supply of blood rich in oxygen to the brain.

Food nourishes the brain and nervous system with the nutrients we need to transform our own enzymes and proteins into the amino acids required to regulate nerve transmission. Those who are very irritable, edgy, and restless, and who suffer wide mood swings between exhilaration and depression, are often suffering from hyperglycemia, too much sugar in the blood. In contrast, starchy foods have a calming effect because they help the body release insulin and aid in the synthesis of one of the brain's important chemicals, seratonin, which regulates mood, appetite, and sleep.

How to control mood swings

Many nutritionists believe our behavior is governed by the foods we eat. We know, for example, that many hyperactive children behave in the way they do because they are reacting adversely to certain foods, so it follows that foods can affect moods. Below are listed various foods that are recommended for boosting the spirits or calming the mind.

Controlling anger and aggression
Eat carbohydrates, including sugar and starch.

Lifting the spirits
Both chilies and spinach are said to raise the spirits.

Relieving tension
Ginger, either in other food or as a drink, has a very calming, soothing effect on frayed nerves.

Relieving winter depression (SAD)
Complex carbohydrates, such as dried beans, pasta, vegetables, and bread.

Staying alert
Protein-rich foods, such as peanuts, chicken, fish, and dried beans.

Improve memory
Liver, fortified cereals and whole grains, as well as zinc-containing foods such as fish. All help as they contain thiamine, riboflavin, beta carotene, and iron.

Aphrodisiacs

Many people put their trust in the power of food to help them attract their partners or to indulge fully in the pleasures of the body. Many strange foods have been thought to invoke passion. The ancient Greeks used rosemary to invigorate and stimulate sexual feelings; the Mexicans and Italians believe basil to be not only an aphrodisiac but also able to increase the size of the male sexual organ. Tomatoes are called love apples in Italy and Spain, but whether they work as an aphrodisiac or not, they are still an excellent source of vitamin C.

Today we can approach the subject of aphrodisiacs more scientifically. For example, we know that peanuts contain histidine, an amino acid the body needs to make histamine, which is important for achieving orgasm. Vitamin E is thought to boost sex drive and fertility because it is known to stimulate the pituitary gland to send out instructions for the release of sex hormones. Some good sources for this sexy vitamin are asparagus, avocados, spinach, olives, nuts, oats, vegetable oils, and whole grains.

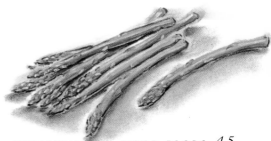

Refreshing Liquids

How healthy is tap water?

As water's vital role in our health is more widely recognized, concern over the level of pollutants in tap water has dramatically increased. There are minerals and chemicals in our drinking water that have been added for various reasons, although some occur naturally. Ammonia and chlorine are added to kill dangerous bacteria, but can also cause dry and irritated skin. Fluoride is added to help prevent tooth decay but this, too, is not good for our skin.

Pesticides and insecticides get into the water system by runoff from the fields, carrying residues into rivers and streams. Some pesticides have chemical substances that mimic the action of the estrogen hormone, and a growing number of researchers are linking the rise in male infertility to the rise in the amount of pesticides flowing into our water.

Is it any wonder that sales of bottled mineral and spring water have increased dramatically? But we shouldn't assume that all bottled water is pure and safe. Natural mineral water, which comes from a natural spring free from pollutants and parasites, is not necessarily safer and is not subject to the same health regulations as tap water. Some may still contain high levels of pesticides and nitrates, depending on the rocks and soil through which the spring water passes.

In fact, surveys have shown that when it comes to comparing bottled still waters, whether mineral, spring, or table water, to filtered tap water, bottled water in many cases was no safer. Bottled still water can contain bacteria, albeit in levels unlikely to do any harm. When the chemicals are filtered from tap water it does not differ much in taste from bottled water.

The main extra ingredient in bottled water seems to be expense. Tap water costs virtually nothing and filtering at home does not significantly raise its cost. Bottled water is considerably more expensive. Some brands of bottled water are nothing more than water straight from a municipal water supply filtered and treated with ultraviolet light and then bottled. So, read the labels on your water bottles and make your choice—or filter your tap water at home.

Water is the great elixir of life. Our bodies, like the planet, contain around 70 percent water. We cannot survive without it—our very core temperature is regulated by the liquid we drink and we would burn up or dry up without it.

In hot countries we tend to drink more water because large amounts of it pass out of the body through sweating and we need to keep our fluid intake up to avoid dehydration. However, in colder countries we tend to drink more than is needed to quench thirst and this surplus leaves the body in the urine. Water not only helps us regulate our temperature, it is also a powerful internal cleanser, dissolving and eliminating waste material to prevent toxicity. It is vital to the body's ability to absorb the nutrients from our food and to replenish lost moisture. Experts recommend that we drink at least eight glasses of water a day. A large intake of water is essential for people on high-fiber diets; they should drink at least the recommended amount if they want to prevent intestinal problems, particularly constipation.

Purifying water

Water is the most recycled product we use. Although vast amounts of money have been spent to clean up our tap water and there have been some real improvements, we can still assume that it is not always perfectly pure, and in fact may be questionably safe. The quality of tap water is a problem throughout the world. In Britain, for example, Friends of the Earth took the government to court several times in the 1980s and 1990s because of drinking water that failed to meet European quality standards.

One way we can clean up our water is by using water filters. These are becoming increasingly popular—the sale of water filters and bottled water began rising dramatically in the late 1980s. Most filters work on the principle of passing water through activated carbon and ion-exchange resins to remove impurities such as lead, nitrates, and other pesticides and herbicides. There is a wide selection of water filters available now and they are very effective, provided the filter is changed regularly. Filters can also be directly connected to the plumbing, and although they are much more expensive, they are also much less bother.

Regardless of which filter system you choose, always be sure to read and follow all instructions to the letter. If you don't, you could make your water quality much worse. Change your filter cartridges frequently. Keep your water jug or container clean and keep filtered water in the refrigerator. Always boil water used for babies' food or drink. When in doubt, particularly when traveling out of the country, always boil the water before drinking if bottled water is not available.

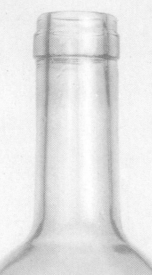

How safe is alcohol?

Almost all celebratory occasions in life involve alcohol. It is associated with pleasure and enjoyment but, as usual, too much of a good thing can be bad for us–and too much alcohol is very bad, causing heart disease, cirrhosis of the liver, and disorders of the stomach and nervous system, not to mention the effect it has on the drinker's family, work, social life, and state of mind.

On the plus side, moderate drinking of red wine is considered good for health and may help protect against heart and lung disease. This theory is based on research carried out in wine-drinking countries such as France and Italy, where the populations regularly tend to drink red wine, rather than white; the red-wine drinkers experience far fewer heart attacks than those who rarely drink wine at all.

Some recent research has suggested that it might not just be red wine but any alcoholic drink taken in moderation that has a health benefit. Moderation means one or two glasses of wine a day, or the equivalent, for maximum protective effect. However, it is best to abstain from alcohol entirely during pregnancy.

Ten herbal teas to try

Herbal teas are a healthy, refreshing, and therapeutic alternative to the tannin- and caffeine-containing tea and coffee we habitually drink. A soothing herbal tea will take the rough edges off a harrowing day while a refreshing one can be the pick-me-up we all need occasionally.

Herbal teas are made from the leaves, flowers, and sometimes the roots of a plant. Drink organic herbal teas regularly for their rich nutrients and to redress and restore balance in the body, maintain strength, prevent degenerative conditions, and accelerate healing.

Making an herbal tea
Pour off-the-boil water over 1 to 2 teaspoons per cup of fresh or dried herbs. Infuse for 5 to 10 minutes. Readymade herbal tea bags are also available.

Borage
This cooling, sweet herb can uplift the spirits and help you cope with a depressive mood. A useful tea for treating colds with fever and bad coughs.

Chamomile
A calming tea that soothes a sensitive stomach or bedtime wakefulness. Good for indigestion, poor appetite, and nervous energy. It helps relieve stress and insomnia.

Elder flower
A sweet, cool, very astringent tea that is often used to prevent or treat colds, flu, hay fever, and other respiratory problems. It encourages sweating and reduces catarrh.

Ginger
Ginger has antinausea and anti-inflammatory effects. It helps alleviate the symptoms of arthritis and is thought to have blood-thinning properties. It also protects against migraine headaches and is said to be a tonic and a mood lifter.

Lemon balm
Lemon balm has a calming effect and is reputed to bring a good night's sleep. It is also recommended for menstrual cramps and for promoting sweating when treating fevers and flu. The leaves have been used for centuries to soothe the digestion and nervous stomachs and to relieve gas.

Marjoram
This is an astringent, warming, and slightly bitter herb that can help soothe asthma attacks, coughs, and indigestion. It is also a useful remedy in the prevention and treatment of menstrual cramps.

Peppermint
Excellent for indigestion and halitosis, peppermint can also help reduce fevers and the symptoms of motion sickness. Mix with lavender to treat migraine headaches.

Rose hip
An infusion of rose hips acts as a general tonic and a mild diuretic and can help relieve the symptoms of a cold.

Rosemary
A bitter, pungent, warming herb and a natural antiseptic. Also used for preventing and treating colds, flu, fatigue, headaches, indigestion, depression, and rheumatism.

Sage
Used to help alleviate symptoms of a sore throat, catarrh, tonsillitis, and laryngitis, sage also has beneficial properties when used to treat indigestion, constipation, and diarrhea if these problems are due to an infection.

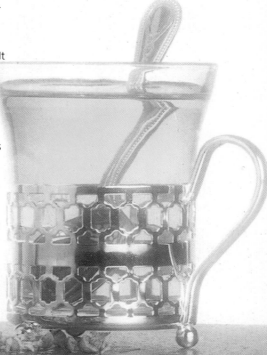

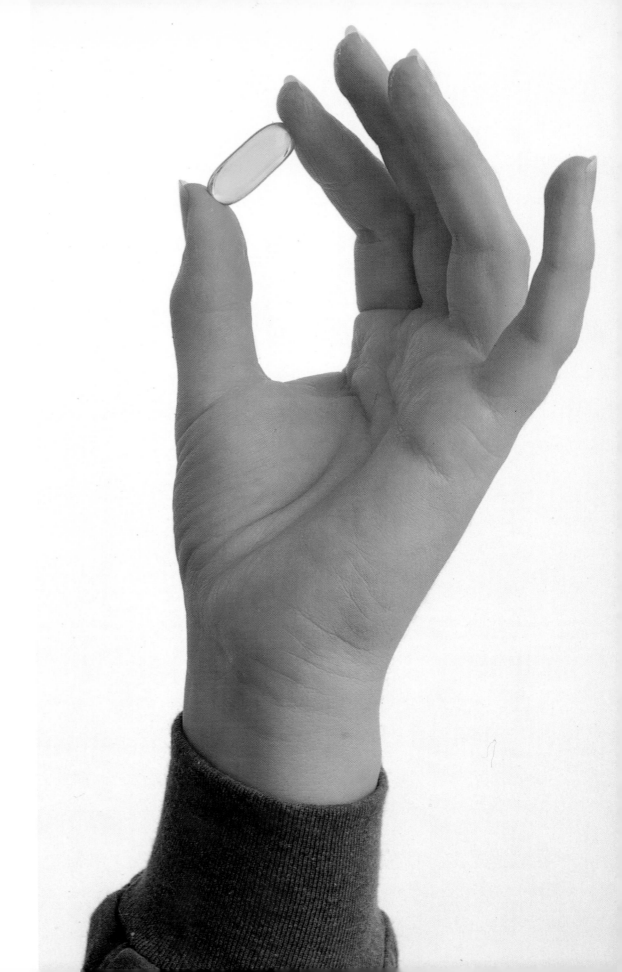

48

3
Dietary Supplements

Vitamins and minerals are the basic, vital nutrients that provide us with life-giving sustenance. We cannot live without them in the same way that we cannot live without air to breathe or water to drink. If we all ate a perfectly balanced diet of fresh, pesticide-free, organically grown food, consumed alcohol in moderation, were always happy and never stressed or ill, we would not need to take any kind of supplement. But life isn't like that. There are times when we need supplements, for example, when recovering from illness, when pregnant, or when we go through menopause. Sometimes we may also need a herbal tonic or some other kind of natural pick-me-up to return us to top form.

The debate on the value of supplements continues to rage. How much, how often, and why are questions hotly debated by the medical profession. You may be advised by your doctor or a nutrition expert to take supplements or you may decide for yourself that you need them. The only way to make a decision is to listen to your body and consult with your practitioner.

What and How Much?

There is no doubt that vitamins and minerals are essential to life and if we all ate a healthy, nutritious, well-balanced diet we would have no need for supplements. Or would we? Many doctors and nutritionists believe in the value of supplements to restore health after illness, disease and immune deficiency conditions. However, even when we are in a good state of health we still need to ensure that we are eating the right foods to gain a sufficient intake of vitamins and minerals.

Governments throughout the world set levels of recommended daily allowances (RDAs), which vary widely from country to country, depending on factors such as dietary habits, availability of local foodstuffs, and even the different types of soil the food is grown in. But these levels are not designed to create optimum health—they are designed to impart information for preventing nutrient deficiency and the many diseases that may result.

It is much more difficult than we realize to eat a diet that meets RDA levels. Even when we are very conscientious about eating a well-balanced diet, we can fall well short of the mark. One survey, carried out in 1985, found that more than 85 percent of people who believed their diet was well balanced failed to meet the recommended levels. Some nutritionists believe that even if these levels were doubled they would still not be high enough in some cases. Others believe that our individual needs and circumstances have a great effect on our nutritional requirements. Patrick Holford, a well-known British nutrition teacher and founder of the Institute for Optimum Nutrition, supports the view that meeting individual needs is not possible using government guidelines. One study tested thousands of people to determine the level of vitamin B in their blood. More than 7 in every 10 people tested were deficient.

If you drink alcohol, smoke, live in the center of a polluted city, or you are pregnant, premenstrual, taking a contraceptive pill, or menopausal—or are experiencing a particularly stressful time—your nutritional needs can easily double.

In another study, done in this country over a 15-year period, 13,500 people were monitored for their nutritional intake. The study found the intake of nutrients associated with optimum health was many times higher than RDA levels. The healthiest were those eating a nutritionally rich diet and taking vitamin and mineral supplements far exceeding government recommendations. This led to the establishment of new guidelines called SONAs (Suggested Optimal Nutrient Allowances) to promote the idea of achieving and maintaining optimal health, rather than suggesting intake levels that will merely ensure we will not get a deficiency disease.

The supplement debate

Synthetic vitamins and minerals are considered useless—or worse, toxic—by some nutritional therapists who advise that natural, organic supplements are the only ones to consider. Of course the purists believe even these are quite worthless and harmful and that fresh, raw fruits and vegetables contain most of our nutritional requirements in their healthiest and most accessible state.

Other nutritionists believe that those who live at a very fast pace, experience a lot of stress, who have limited access to fresh fruits and vegetables, who drink alcohol, or smoke require at least double the usual amount of nutrients. Environmental pollution, "sick" buildings, whether we are male or female, young or old—all these factors influence our very individual vitamin and mineral requirements.

There is, however, unanimous agreement in one area only and that is that eating more fresh, raw, and organic (pesticide-free) fruits and vegetables is a great booster to better health and a strong sense of well-being.

The choice of supplements in a health food store can be bewildering. If you have some idea of what you want, such as an antioxidant preparation to combat free radicals in the body (released both by the body's own natural processes and as a consequence of air pollution) the choice should be simple. Similarly, a B-complex preparation should not be too hard to find. But perhaps the simplest thing to do if you think you need more minerals and vitamins is to take a one-a-day combined multivitamin and multimineral preparation. Generally, the amounts of substances contained in it will be comfortably above the recommended daily figures but will not be high enough to cause any problems.

Recommended daily allowances (U.S.) (Based on 2,000 calories per day)		
Vitamin	**Male**	**Female**
A (Beta carotene)	5,000 IU	4,000 IU
B_1	1.5 mg	1.1 mg
B_2	1.7 mg	1.3-1.6 mg
B_3	19 mg	15-17 mg
B_5	4-7 mg	4-7 mg
B_6	2 mg	1.6-2.2 mg
B_{12}	2 mcg	2-2.2 mcg
Folic acid	200 mcg	180-400 mcg
PABA	No set figure	
Biotin	30-100 mcg	30-100 mcg
C	60 mg	60-70 mg
D	200 IU	200-400 IU
E	15 IU	12-15 IU
K	80 mcg	65 mcg

Reading the labels

Supplement labels: Choosing vitamin and mineral supplements can be confusing. The key is to understand the labels. Information is usually explained on the packaging, since supplements come in pill or capsule form. It should show the amount per dose, sometimes accompanied by how much that dose is as a percentage of the recommended daily allowance, or percent Daily Value (expressed as % DV). But the numbers and units used for the weights of a mineral or vitamin can be baffling. There is a simple logic to it, however. The weights given are in the metric system and thus "g" stands for "gram," "mg" means "milligram" (1/1,000 of a gram), and "mcg" means "microgram" (1/1,000,000 of a gram). For some supplements, the RDA is given "IU," meaning "international units" (vitamin D 400 IU, for example).

Figuring out the nutritional value of supplements has become easier. The FDA requires that supplements packaged after July of 1995 must include the percent Daily Value (% DV), instead of the RDA. So look for the % DV figures and you'll know instantly the value of the vitamins and minerals you are getting in each dose. It is best to take a multivitamin, multimineral supplement packaged by a large, reputable company. As a rule, supplements of this sort should contain 100% of the RDA, or Daily Value. One Centrum tablet taken daily, for example, will provide 5,000 IU of vitamin A (40% as beta carotene), or 100% DV, and 15 mg (100% DV) of the micromineral zinc. Among all the other vitamins and minerals provided, one tablet also provides 20 mcg of selenium, which is shown as an asterisk in the % DV column because the RDA for selenium has not been determined.

Food labels: If you want to work out how much of a vitamin or mineral you are getting in frozen, canned, prepared, and packaged foods, first look for the Nutrition Facts box on the label. Below the listings for calories, total fat, saturated fat, cholesterol, sodium, carbohydrates (fiber and sugars), and protein, you will find the % DV for some of the vitamins and minerals in that food. If you are want to figure out how much vitamin A you are getting, for example, a serving of canned, cooked sweet potatoes in corn syrup might provide 230% DV of vitamin A (100% as beta carotene) and a serving of solid white tuna packed in water 0% DV of vitamin A. But the tuna label will also tell you that you are getting 10% DV of vitamin B_6, 15% DV of vitamin B_{12}, and 10% DV of phosphorus in that serving. (Fresh foods are generally not sold with this sort of information and vitamin and mineral content will vary with the freshness of the produce, the soil it was grown in, etc.)

Vitamins

Vitamins are complex organic substances found in minute amounts in the food we eat and, in the case of vitamin D, additionally provided by sunlight. They ensure proper growth and development and healthy body maintenance while also actively controlling how our bodies make use of other nutrients. Any deficiencies can alter the nutritional intake of the body and may lead to illness. However, excessive doses of some vitamins can be just as harmful as deficiencies—vitamins A and D particularly can build up in the body to toxic levels.

There is no doubt that occasionally we need to replace depleted levels of vitamins in the body. If you decide to take supplements, stick to the recommended dosages. Any increases in this dose should only be taken if recommended by a doctor. Never give supplements to infants or children without a doctor's advice.

Vitamin A (Retinol)

Vitamin A promotes good vision, skin, and hair. It helps keep the digestive system healthy and is necessary for proper growth and formation of the teeth and bones. It is important not to take too much of this vitamin because it can reach toxic levels.

Natural sources:
Fish liver oils, liver, butter, eggs, cheese and milk, carrots, tomatoes, spinach, broccoli, winter squash, lettuce, green and red peppers, apricots, cantaloupe, and mangoes.

When more might help:
Vitamin A can boost the immune system and might be helpful if suffering from cancer, measles, or respiratory infections. It might also be beneficial for those suffering gastric ulcers, acne, eczema, or psoriasis. Extra vitamin A might be needed if large amounts of alcohol are consumed.

Daily dose:
Pregnant women should seek medical advice before taking supplements of vitamin A. Do not take a supplement if you are also taking beta carotene in a supplement. A typical dose is 4,000 to 5,000 IU a day in a multivitamin pill. Doses should not exceed 5,000 IU daily.

Beta carotene

The body easily converts this nutrient into vitamin A. The high intake of natural beta carotene is thought to protect against the development of cancer and heart disease since it protects against cell damage and inhibits the activity of free radicals in the body.

Natural sources:
Fruits and vegetables, especially yellow and orange ones, e.g. carrots.

When more might help:
If you smoke; and to prevent artery disease, otherwise as for vitamin A.

Supplement dose:
15 mg daily. Often found as part of an anti-oxidant multivitamin with vitamin C and vitamin E.

Vitamin B$_1$ (Thiamine)

Important for a healthy nervous system, B$_1$ is needed for the release of energy from food for growth and energy production. It helps burn calories. This vitamin prevents beriberi–a deficiency linked to depression, sleep disturbances, chronic fatigue, mental confusion, digestive problems, anemia, an impaired immune system, water retention, muscle weakness, and even heart failure and lung damage. Vitamin B$_1$ is destroyed by alcohol and is easily attacked by environmental factors.

Natural sources:
Wheat germ, whole grains, soybeans, brown rice, whole-grain pasta, bran, pumpernickel bread, brewer's yeast, potatoes, Brazil nuts, pecans, cashews, peanuts, pork, liver, milk, eggs, peas, and orange and grapefruit juice.

When more might help:
A deficiency might be caused by the following: a high alcohol intake, eating a lot of raw fish, eating a high-carbohydrate diet (especially "empty calories"), or long-term use of antacids. Extra B$_1$ might help during pregnancy and breast-feeding, if suffering from diabetes, when under stress, during a fever, after surgery, or for those with a raised metabolic rate, such as hyperthyroidism.

Daily dose:
Most well-balanced diets contain enough thiamine but it can be taken as a supplement, usually as part of a B-complex or multivitamin preparation. A typical supplement dose found in such preparations is between 1.5 and 1.9 mg.

Vitamin B$_2$ (Riboflavin)

Contributes considerably to enzyme activity that controls the chemical reactions in the body, including digestion, where it helps the body use the calories in food. It helps convert proteins, fats, and carbohydrates into energy important for growth, including maintaining healthy eyes, mouth, and skin. Riboflavin influences the production of hormones by the adrenal glands and is essential for cell growth.

Natural sources:
Cheese, eggs, breakfast cereals, liver, kidneys, almonds, green vegetables, and avocados.

When more might help:
If you get only moderate amounts of exercise, drink alcohol, smoke, or are on the contraceptive pill. A supplement might also be of use if you take diuretics, tricyclic drugs, or antidepressants. Diabetics and pregnant or breast-feeding women may need more.

Daily dose:
Most people get enough riboflavin in their diets but if you need more, it can be taken in a multivitamin supplement or in a B-complex tablet. A daily dose between 1.7 and 2 mg is sufficient.

Vitamin B$_3$ (Niacin, Nicotinic Acid)

An important catalyst for the release of energy from carbohydrates, protein, and fat in food along with thiamine and riboflavin. Niacin can almost be divided into two parts: The acid form is connected with the circulatory system, maintenance of the nervous system, and reducing fats and cholesterol levels. The other part of niacin helps break down protein, carbohydrates, and fats. It also helps the body produce energy and release energy from food.

Natural sources:
Chicken, beef, eggs, liver, lamb, tuna, swordfish, salmon, oysters, almonds, peanuts and other nuts, beans, and whole-grain bread.

When more might help:
The average diet contains only about half of the optimal amount of vitamin B$_3$ (19 mg). As with other B-vitamins, those who drink large amounts of alcohol might need more. Pregnant and breast-feeding women, those who get little exercise or are on antileukemia drugs should ensure they get enough.

Daily dose:
More than 2,000 mg daily is toxic. Take as part of a multivitamin or as a B-complex formulation–20 mg is a typical dose.

Vitamin B$_5$ (Pantothenic Acid)

In supplement form it is often referred to as calcium pantothenate. It is part of the coenzyme A molecule, which plays a major part in the process of energy release from the food you eat. It is also very important for the formation of antibodies and for the healthy functioning of the adrenal glands.

Natural sources:
Brewer's yeast, liver, nuts, bran, wheat germ, eggs, and poultry.

When more might help:
Stress or taking antibiotics might call for more, as might eating a diet low in fresh food (processing can remove a lot of B$_3$). Diabetics and those who consume large amounts of alcohol might need more.

Daily dose:
Take as part of a multivitamin or as a B-complex formulation–4 to 10 mg daily is enough. Doses over 10 g may cause diarrhea.

Vitamin B$_6$ (Pyridoxine)

Converts quickly into coenzymes, which play a vital role in protein metabolism, fat metabolism, energy, and hemoglobin production. This vitamin also has an effect on activity in the central nervous system. Pyridoxine is also involved in the metabolism of amino acids, nucleic acids, and glycogen. It helps regulate hormone balance, red blood cells, and the nervous and immune systems. Some diabetics and people with certain food intolerances have responded well to vitamin B$_6$ therapy.

Natural sources:
Wheat germ, turkey, chicken, whitefish, beef, potatoes, Brussels sprouts, bananas, peas, beans, lentils, broccoli, cauliflower.

When more might help:
Despite the wide availability in food many people do not get enough vitamin B$_6$, even though they consume a sufficient amount to avoid deficiency symptoms. A supplement might be a good idea when taking the contraceptive pill or if pregnant or breast-feeding. Too much alcohol and smoking are also signs that a supplement might help. A high-protein diet can also mean that the body may need more B$_6$.

Daily dose:
Doses over 500 mg are toxic and can cause nerve damage. Some drugs interfere with the way the body eliminates B$_6$, including hydralazine, isoniazid, and penicillamine, which is used to treat rheumatoid arthritis, so always seek a doctor's advice. The general rule is never take more than 50 mg per day. Take as part of a multivitamin or as a B-complex formulation.

Vitamin B$_{12}$

The essential vitamin for a healthy nervous system, red blood cells, and bone marrow. It is a very important vitamin for maintaining and preventing damage to the nervous system, is essential for the formation of new cells, particularly red blood cells, and helps to prevent or treat anemia. It is needed for the synthesis of DNA, the metabolism of fatty acids, and for keeping the myelin sheath around the nerves healthy. B$_{12}$ particularly works in tandem with folic acid and needs a substance present in gastric juice, or intrinsic factor, to be absorbed by your body.

Natural sources:
Found in foods of animal origin–such as liver, kidney, meat, fish, eggs, cheese–and in brewer's yeast.

When more might help:
As B$_{12}$ is almost exclusively found in animal food sources, vegans or strict vegetarians may need more. Supplements might help in old age, during pregnancy, and breast-feeding. Heavy alcohol drinkers or smokers may need more. Certain drugs can also lower the body's B$_{12}$ levels, so check with your doctor if you are receiving medication for an existing condition.

Daily dose:
Take as part of a multivitamin or B-complex preparation–3 to 4 mcg daily is recommended.

Folic Acid (Vitamin B₉)

This is part of the B-complex vitamin group and is needed for many physiological reactions, such as the synthesis of DNA and for cell division. It helps the production of genetic material inside the cells, and like the other B vitamins, folic acid helps to maintain a healthy nervous system. This nutrient is vital before conception and during pregnancy. There is strong evidence that folic acid supplements before pregnancy and in its early stages can prevent spina bifida and neural defects.

Natural sources:
Wheat germ, brewer's yeast, green leafy vegetables like spinach and watercress, whole-grain and whole-wheat bread and cereal, chicken liver, and nuts.

When more might help:
Folic acid benefits those planning to become pregnant, those who are pregnant, breast-feeding mothers, heavy alcohol drinkers, elderly people, and those on an estrogen-containing contraceptive pill. Some drugs make it difficult for the body to absorb folic acid, so check with your doctor. It has been shown to have some protective effect against cancer and might help protect against heart disease.

Daily dose:
Take as part of a multivitamin preparation. Doses are between 180 and 400 mcg. Pregnant women or those who might become pregnant should take 400 mcg per day. Do not take more than 1,500 mcg per day.

PABA (Para-Aminobenzoic Acid)

This nutrient is part of the structure of folic acid rather than a true vitamin in its own right. It has some involvement in the metabolism of amino acids and red blood cells. PABA is a common ingredient in sunscreens. It is best taken with the other B-complex vitamins.

Natural sources:
Wheat germ, molasses, eggs, and liver.

When more might help:
Under medical supervision to treat vitiligo and other skin complaints.

Daily dose:
Usually applied in a sunscreen preparation or taken orally under medical supervision. It is found in B-complex preparations. Sustained megadosing can damage liver, kidneys, and heart.

Biotin (Vitamin B₇, Vitamin H)

The eighth and final B vitamin operates with the rest of the B-complex vitamins to affect the metabolism of carbohydrates, energy, and fat. Biotin is important in fat and glycogen manufacture. Some nutritionists recommend biotin supplements for treating candida albicans to prevent the condition's worsening into its fungal form.

Natural sources:
Brewer's yeast, bran, wheat germ, eggs, chicken, liver, and kidney.

When more might help:
People under stress and those taking antibiotics or antibacterial drugs from the sulfonamide group might need more biotin. Pregnant or breast-feeding women should ensure they get enough either through their diet or with a supplement.

Daily dose:
It is found in multi- and B-complex preparations in a dose of 30 to 100 mcg.

Vitamin C (Ascorbic Acid)

This vital vitamin is one of the "super vitamins." It acts as a powerful antioxidant, effectively neutralizing free radicals, the highly destructive chemical substances that change or destroy healthy cells and that many experts believe are the basis of many serious degenerative conditions, including heart disease and cancer. White blood cells contain a generous amount of vitamin C and are the body's main fighters against invading germs. Vitamin C needs to be taken daily–the body cannot store it. Smokers need more vitamin C. It is important for healthy bones, teeth, and gums, as well as for fighting infection. It helps maintain the skin and is important in the formation of collagen for tissue repair, for growth, and for the healing of wounds. Vitamin C helps the body absorb iron, metabolize folic acid, form antibodies, and stimulate the white blood cells. There is some evidence that large doses help prevent the common cold. The body does not manufacture or store this vitamin, hence the importance of fresh, raw fruits and vegetables rich in vitamin C. Studies have shown women whose diets are the highest in vitamin C foods are at the lowest risk for breast cancer. This vitamin is crucial for energy–and even for our breathing and heartbeat.

Natural sources:
Raw fruits and vegetables–citrus fruits, black currants, tomatoes, green leafy vegetables, mangoes, green pepper–and Brussels sprouts, sweet potatoes, potatoes.

When more might help:
This is an essential vitamin and we should ensure we get enough of it. Those who may need supplements include the elderly, diabetics, pregnant or breast-feeding women, those taking the contraceptive pill, people who have had a serious injury or surgery, who are chronically ill, and those exposed to environmental pollution, especially vehicle exhaust. And, of course, those who drink to excess and smoke. The vitamin is thought also to be protective against heart and artery disease and certain types of cancer, especially cancers of the cervix, lung, breast, mouth, throat, stomach, pancreas, colon, and rectum. It is also thought to help back pain and help prevent cataracts. Some nutritionists believe that extra vitamin C can help increase a low sperm count.

Daily dose:
A reasonable supplement dose would

be between 60 mg and 70 mg per day. Up to 1,000 mg is safe.

Vitamin D (Calciferol)

This fat-soluble vitamin is very important for children, who need greater quantities of D for their fast-growing, developing bones. Deficiency signs include skeletal deformity, painful bones and muscle weakness, tenderness in the pelvis, spine, shoulders, and ribs. Our body converts vitamin D to a hormone that controls calcium function and absorption. It is formed in the skin when the body is exposed to sunlight, and it is vital for the bones' ability to absorb calcium and phosphorus.

Natural sources:
Mostly in dairy and animal products and particularly in cod-liver oil, herring, canned salmon, eggs, milk, butter, and margarine.

When more might help:
Taking more might help when there is low exposure to sunshine and when animal foodstuffs are not in the diet. Vitamin D protects against osteoporosis. The elderly might need more, as might heavy drinkers, women who are breast-feeding or pregnant, people with liver or kidney diseases, those taking anticonvulsants, mineral oil, or cholesterol-reducing compounds.

Daily dose:
A daily dose of 400 to 600 IU should be enough. It can be found in single-ingredient and multivitamin preparations. Vitamin D can be highly toxic, especially to fetuses and children. Consult a doctor.

Vitamin E (Alpha-Tocopherol)

The fat-soluble vitamin E is a member of the powerful antioxidant family that keeps the molecules in the blood and tissues from becoming damaged by oxidation. Vitamin E is reputed to slow down cell aging, help repair the skin, and promote growth and the formation of new blood cells. Its positive antioxidant effect also helps prevent degeneration of the nerves and muscles. Vitamin E is considered the fertility and heart vitamin. It also stimulates healing and helps prevent atherosclerosis and thrombosis. Some of the conditions vitamin E is reputed to help include circulatory problems, fibrocystic breast conditions, heart disease, Parkinson's disease, PMS (particularly when taken with evening primrose oil), and thrombosis.

Natural sources:
Wheat-germ oil, safflower and sunflower oils, sunflower seeds, almonds, whole-grain cereals, wheat germ, margarine, peanut butter, green leafy vegetables, and asparagus.

When more might help:
Women who are breast-feeding or pregnant might need more vitamin E, as might smokers and heavy drinkers. If you consume a large amount of polyunsaturated fats such as corn oil, sunflower oil, and safflower oil you will need more, as will those who have to breathe polluted air. People suffering from cystic fibrosis, pancreatitis, Crohn's disease, and liver disease may need more. Those taking mineral oil and cholesterol-lowering drugs might benefit from a supplement. Vitamin E is said to protect against cancer and diseases of the heart and arteries. It is also thought to boost the immune system, reduce the likelihood of cataracts, and slow down the onset of Parkinson's.

Daily dose:
Vitamin E supplements are found alone and in combination. A daily dose is 30 to 40 IU. Doses over 2,400 IU cause excess bleeding.

Vitamin K

An important vitamin that helps the body form the proteins necessary for blood clotting. Bacteria in the digestive system provide half the required amount of this vitamin. Deficiency may manifest itself in nose bleeds or excessive bleeding.

Natural sources:
Mostly in a few vegetables such as Brussels sprouts, cabbage, cauliflower, and spinach.

When more might help:
When long-term antibiotics are used and for those suffering from jaundice. Those with liver disease, ulcerative colitis, and Crohn's disease might have a deficiency.

Daily dose:
Not usually necessary. Excess vitamin K can cause brain damage in infants.

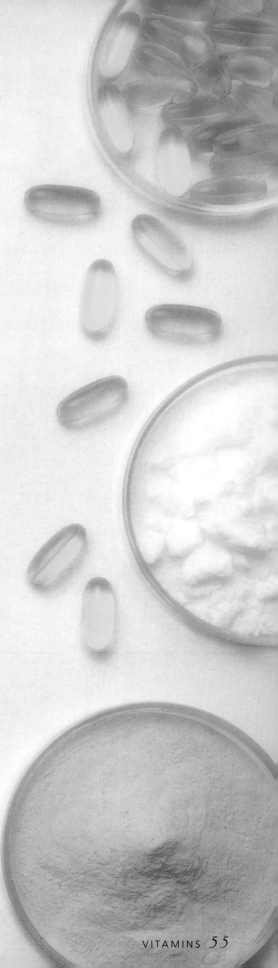

Minerals

Minerals are the essential building blocks of all living matter. They are found in the Earth's crust and make their way into the sea, soil, and groundwater. From there, minerals get into the fruits, vegetables, and grains that are then consumed by both animals and humans.

A balanced mineral intake is essential to keeping well and preventing the development of disease. Recent research suggests that the role minerals play in our continued well-being is crucial and often underestimated. They are vital to our ability to maintain health and avoid illness. Our bodies need minerals to absorb and utilize vitamins, enzymes, and amino acids and also to build healthy new cells. Some experts now believe degenerative disease may be due to mineral deficiencies that cause cell breakdown.

There are seven major minerals, also known as the macrominerals, of which we need a substantial amount—more than 100 mg a day—to keep our body function healthy. The other important minerals are known as trace elements or microminerals, because we need only tiny amounts, or traces, of them.

Mineral supplements are not to be taken lightly or without thought; some are toxic when taken to excess, especially some of the trace elements. Undue use of minerals can throw the body off balance and might do more harm than good. If in any doubt, or if you are taking medication, check with your doctor or with a qualified nutritionist. Otherwise take a balanced, organic multimineral supplement made by a well-established, reputable company.

Macrominerals

Calcium
The most abundant mineral in the body, calcium is very important for building strong bones and teeth and for maintaining bone density and strength in later life. Women at risk from osteoporosis (thinning of the bones leading to easy breaks and fractures) are usually advised to eat more calcium-rich food and in many cases to take supplements.

Calcium also helps the blood clot properly. Together with phosphorus, calcium also helps the easy movement of our muscles. Calcium helps metabolize iron, regulates the heart, and alleviates nervous stress and insomnia. Calcium also has many special prevention features—it protects the body from heavy metal poisoning, particularly lead and cadmium, and also any environmental pollutants that challenge the immune system.
Natural sources:
Green leafy vegetables, such as spinach, cabbage, and watercress; pumpkin; root vegetables; raisins and figs; milk, powdered milk, cheese, and yogurt; soybeans and tofu; sesame, sunflower, and pumpkin seeds; and salmon and sardines (with the bones).

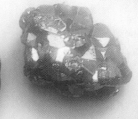
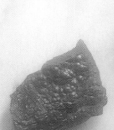

When more might help:
To help prevent osteoporosis. Taken in combination with magnesium and potassium, it can help prevent high blood pressure and intestinal cancer. It can also help lower blood cholesterol levels.

Low levels of calcium are found in some very serious conditions, particularly osteoporosis. In the United States more than 24 million people–80 percent of them women–suffer from this illness, which causes major bone loss, rendering sufferers prone to fractures. In the U.S. about 1.3 million fractures are attributed to osteoporosis each year. About one-third of elderly women with hip fractures die within six months.

Supplement dose:
500 mg calcium and 250 mg magnesium combined a day. It is a good idea to take extra vitamin C when taking a calcium supplement.

Chloride
Provides the chloride for hydrochloric acid in the stomach, so helps the digestion. Helps maintain fluid levels in the body. Contributes to healthy hair and teeth. Chloride is found in numerous foodstuffs, and is a major component of common salt.

Natural sources:
Salt, kelp, yogurt, and olives.

When more might help:
During heavy sweating.

Supplement dose:
Salt tablets only in very hot climates.

Magnesium
This mineral works in tandem with calcium–each needs the other to function fully. It also helps convert blood sugar into energy. Magnesium is important for developing the bones and for maintaining muscles and nerves. It is an essential mineral for the healthy transmission of nerve impulses, for relaxing the muscles, and for countless other body functions–from the functioning of DNA to our body's enzyme activity. One of nature's natural tranquilizers, magnesium is often called the antistress nutrient. In supplement form it is best taken in a balanced multimineral supplement that also includes calcium, phosphorus, and potassium.

Natural sources:
Green vegetables–particularly dark leafy ones like spinach–apples, figs, grapefruit and lemons, sesame seeds, peanuts, peas and beans, seafood, whole-grain bread and cereals, and tropical fruit.

When more might help:
A steady balance of calcium and magnesium can help prevent and treat stress, depression, PMS, cramps, and sugar cravings. Can also help with sleeplessness.

Supplement dose:
250 to 400 mg a day combined with twice the amount of calcium. Do not take magnesium during pregnancy.

Phosphorus
The most abundant mineral in the body after calcium, phosphorus is found in every cell in the body but stored mainly in the bones and teeth. Very important for cell and tissue repair, phosphorus is essential for the body's ability to produce energy. It is crucial in the prevention of serious stress disorders, joint stiffness, arthritis, and even cancer. It is present in every cell and affects the transfer of nerve impulses. It helps us metabolize fats and starches and plays a role in the regularity of our heart, plus the structure of our bones and teeth. It is very important to have a balanced phosphorus and calcium intake so take the same amounts at a time. Too much phosphorus over calcium can lower calcium performance, leading to low levels of body calcium, which in time can create the conditions for the development of osteoporosis.

Natural sources:
Dairy foods have the most balanced phosphorus and calcium content. Brown rice, lentils, nuts, seeds, beans–particularly mung beans–whole grains, fish, poultry, meat, and eggs are other sources.

When more might help:
This mineral is a nervous system tonic and is often called the mood mineral.

Supplement dose:
Combine 500 mg phosphorus with 500 mg calcium and 250 mg magnesium a day. You may need more, but seek a doctor's advice first.

Potassium
Known as the brain mineral, potassium partly regulates the fluid level in the body, monitoring the balance between water and sodium inside and outside the cells. It helps send oxygen to the brain, get rid of the body's wastes, and reduce blood pressure. It can also be useful in treating allergies and relieving bloating due to water retention. Potassium is very important for nerve impulse transmission and for metabolizing the food we eat into energy. It is crucial to our neuromuscular system and to the healthy functioning of our cardiovascular and nervous systems. If you suffer from hypertension (high blood pressure) or fluid retention, the body is likely to need more potassium and a supplement may be required. Potassium functions in combination with sodium and it is important to maintain a balance between them. This can be a problem since much more sodium (in the form of common salt) is added to processed, packaged, and refined foods, as well as most fast food. Also, potassium is very easily lost through cooking and excretion.

Natural sources:
Raisins, bananas, citrus fruits, avocados, apples, apricots, lettuce, cauliflower, tomatoes, green leafy vegetables, watercress, potatoes, barley, whole grains, dandelion and mint leaves, meat, and poultry.

When more might help:
During severe gastroenteritis, when diarrhea and vomiting deplete the body's stores, or if suffering from muscular weakness or low blood pressure. Keeping our potassium level up is helpful in preventing high blood pressure and strokes. A potassium supplement may help to balance out high sodium levels.

Supplement dose:
An excess may be dangerous for those with heart conditions, so consult a doctor first.

Sodium

The "fluid mineral" regulates the balance of water in the body. It helps prevent heat exhaustion and sunstroke as well as helping in the healthy functioning of nerves and muscles. Salt is 40 percent sodium and 60 percent chloride, so there is little chance of suffering from a sodium deficiency, given our salt-laden modern diet. Only those who do very heavy physical work, such as athletes and manual workers, or those who perspire excessively need to take a supplement. In fact, nearly all foods have some form of sodium and the incidence of high blood pressure in Western countries is partly blamed on our high sodium intake.

Natural sources:
Salt, kelp, beets, figs, coconut, carrots, artichokes, and shellfish.

When more might help:
Only if sweating profusely in hot climates.

Supplement dose:
Take as salt tablets in hot climates.

Sulfur

The purifying mineral is excellent for skin, hair, and nails. It helps keep them healthy and prevents acne. It also helps to fight bacterial infection and to maintain proper liver secretions, such as bile, and brain function.

Natural sources:
Cabbage, dried beans, raspberries, fish, and eggs.

When more might help:
Only strict vegetarians risk deficiency. Unnecessary unless specifically prescribed by a medical practitioner.

Supplement dose:
Found in sufficient foodstuffs to make supplements unnecessary.

Microminerals

Chromium

This trace mineral helps in the body's efficient use of glucose by balancing the output of insulin. Chromium also helps to balance blood sugar levels, hence playing an important part in the prevention of diabetes, high blood pressure, and arteriosclerosis. Chromium also reduces the level of cholesterol in the blood. So much of this mineral is lost during the processing of food that it is difficult to get too much of this important mineral.

Natural sources:
Whole grains, brewer's yeast, mushrooms, legumes, nuts, meat, shellfish, chicken, and corn oil.

When more might help:
If dieting (but only on the advice of a doctor). Might help with high blood pressure.

Supplement dose:
100 mcg a day. Do not take while pregnant or breast-feeding.

Cobalt

This mineral helps to build red blood cells and prevent anemia. It is an essential component of vitamin B_{12}. We get all the cobalt we need from this vitamin.

Natural sources:
Liver, kidney, meat, eggs, milk and dairy products, fish, and enriched cereals.

When more might help:
If on a vegan diet, in old age, if a heavy smoker, if alcohol intake is high.

Supplement dose:
1 mcg a day. Megadoses (20 to 30 mg per day) are dangerous.

Copper

While controlling the action of many enzymes, this trace element is important for blood and bone formation and for protecting skin pigmentation. It is essential for the production of hemoglobin, the molecule that carries the oxygen in the blood. This mineral's presence is also essential for the proper utilization of vitamin C and helps in the absorption of iron. Too much copper can be toxic or lead to anemia.

Natural sources:
Peas, dried beans, mushrooms, prunes, whole grains, shrimp, and liver.

When more might help:
To help prevent rheumatoid arthritis.

1 to 2 mg a day, although not usually needed. Should be taken as part of a balanced supplement only. Seek a doctor's advice.

Fluorine
This is the mineral that strengthens our teeth, bones, and tissues. Flouride, the synthetic version of the mineral, is added to drinking water and toothpastes. It can be highly toxic in large doses.
Natural sources:
Tea, especially China tea; seafood, egg whites, cabbage, radishes, beets, lettuce, garlic, whole wheat, and gelatin.
When more might help:
If living in a region where water is not fluoridated.
Supplement dose:
In a fluoride-containing toothpaste.

Iodine
Promotes a balanced metabolism and burning of excessive fat, promotes growth and energy. It contributes to healthy hair, teeth, and nails and to a positive and lively mental attitude. It plays an important role in the healthy function of the thyroid gland.
Natural sources:
Fish, seaweed, seafood, vegetables grown in rich soil, iodized table salt, and cod-liver oil.
When more might help:
If unable to eat fish or seafood and on low-salt diet.
Supplement dose:
Kelp tablets. Seek medical advice.

Iron
This is a very important trace mineral for the body. It is the blood mineral that is essential to the body's energy-producing functions. It helps form hemoglobin, which carries the vital oxygen within our red blood cells. It is also important in the production of enzymes that regulate metabolism and the absorption of the B vitamins. Muscle activity is affected by iron intake. Tannic acid in tea and coffee blocks the body's absorption of iron. Iron deficiencies are very common, but usually easy to treat.
Natural sources:
Green leafy vegetables, cereals, whole-grain bread, parsley, kelp, brown rice, soybeans, beets, apricots, raisins, oatmeal, liver, red meat, eggs, nuts, and beans.
When more might help:
After loss of blood, if suffering from anemia, during heavy periods, or for women during their childbearing years. It is also advisable if on a meat-free diet. Excessive tea and coffee drinking inhibits the body's absorption of iron.
Supplement dose:
Females in puberty and women during menopause often need a supplement. But sustained use can be toxic, particularly for fetuses, infants, and elderly men. Seek medical advice before taking iron tablets on a long-term basis.

Manganese
Vital for the efficient transmission of nerve impulses. Improves memory, reflexes, and poor digestion, and helps to eliminate fatigue. Calms the nerves and reduces irritability. Manganese helps the body in the synthesis of cholesterol and the sex hormones. It helps in bone and connective tissue formation, metabolizing the proteins and carbohydrates in the body and fats in the blood.
Natural sources:
Whole-grain cereals, seeds, and nuts; some green leafy vegetables, peas, beets, egg yolks, and some tropical fruit and avocados. Also in tea.
When more might help:
To help prevent arteriosclerosis.
Supplement dose:
2 to 4.5 mg a day. Best taken with vitamins B and C to redress the body's balance and build strength. Seek medical advice.

Selenium
This mineral is one of the important antioxidants, helping to protect the cells and delay the signs of aging. It works well with vitamins E and C. There is evidence that it helps protect against cancer. It keeps the liver functioning well and helps maintain the heart. It is also essential for good eyesight and has an anti-inflammatory effect, which helps relieve the symptoms of rheumatoid arthritis. It is also a very important mineral for the male reproductive system and can help alleviate some of the symptoms of menopause. It will help prevent dry skin and dandruff.

Natural sources:
Liver, fish and shellfish, eggs, garlic, broccoli, tomatoes, onions, wheat germ, brown rice, bran, whole grains, and brewer's yeast.
When more might help:
To build immunity, to help with stress, for arthritis and high blood pressure.
Supplement dose:
60 to 70 mcg a day. Never exceed 200 mcg a day from all sources, including food.

Zinc
Necessary for healthy growth and balanced moods. It can help treat impotence and low sex drive, tone the reproductive organs, and aid in the prevention of prostate problems. It also helps reduce cholesterol deposits and maintain the body's acid-alkaline balance. In addition, it plays a part in the formation of insulin, promotes proper brain function, and considerably accelerates the healing process. Zinc is an important component of many enzymes in the digestive and reproductive systems.
Natural sources:
Shellfish, poultry, red meat, eggs, milk, cheese, yogurt, brewer's yeast, wheat germ, pecans, pumpkin seeds, mustard, chilies, and cocoa.
When more might help:
Zinc is useful when the body is fighting infections and helps the healing of wounds. It is good for anemia and when on the contraceptive pill.
Supplement dose:
10 to 20 mg a day. Seek advice before taking larger doses.

Tonics and Elixirs

Virtually all cultures, from Native Americans to the ancient Chinese and from Aboriginal Australians to the Indian tribes of South America, have used the healing powers of herbs and plants to make preparations for restoring tranquillity to the mind, health to the body, and preventing the onset of disease. Probably the most ancient of all medical techniques, the use of herbal tonics, tinctures, elixirs, and herbal teas is becoming an increasingly popular approach in the modern world to restoring energy to a tired body and mind. They are also invaluable when used in the prevention of illness to build up the body's strength and natural resilience. The demands of modern life can make us all feel stressed, tired and in need of a pick-me-up from time to time. Nature has conveniently created a pharmacopoeia of health-giving, natural restoratives that are rapidly gaining in popularity with the general public and health workers worldwide.

Herbal tonics and elixirs are available that will help in preserving and maintaining your vitality and well-being, assist recovery during convalescence, and speed the body's natural healing process during illness. However, do not allow feelings of fatigue, stress or general weakness to continue over a prolonged period without seeking medical advice. Many preparations have been designed for self-help, and a variety of herbal practitioners, working in a range of many international traditions, may also be consulted. There is a long history of herbal medicine in Europe and many preparations are also available from the Hakims found in Asian communities and from Chinese herbalists and practitioners of traditional Chinese medicine. The following tonics are among the most popular.

Aloe
The jellylike liquid of aloe leaves is reputed to have healing properties for both internal and external wounds and for soothing irritated skin. It is an effective preventive or treatment for irritable bowel syndrome and good for the digestive system. Prolonged or excessive use may induce hemorrhoids. Consult a qualified practitioner before taking aloe internally.

Cider vinegar
Cider vinegar tones up the immune system, balances the body's chemistry and helps prevent and treat kidney stones and most arthritic conditions. The usual dosage is one teaspoon mixed with honey and warm water, taken three times a day.

Cod liver oil
This important fish oil is a time-honored favorite for protecting health. A daily dose—one capsule—of this fish oil will tone up your general health and is a valuable source of vitamins A and D.

Coenzyme Q_{10}
Important for the production of energy in the body, this new supplement is often referred to as the wonder vitamin Q. Actually, it is a coenzyme. It enables the body's cells to release energy from food. While the body manufactures this enzyme itself, illness, aging, and generally lowered resistance tend to reduce production. To maintain or boost energy levels take up to three capsules daily. It is not recommended for pregnant or breast-feeding women.

Damiana
This herb has a reputation for rejuvenating the reproductive organs because it increases the blood flow to the capillaries. It also stimulates the genitourinary tract when excreted and so appears to stimulate the sex organs. It may have this effect because it has a nervine action, creating a feeling of mild euphoria for one to two hours. It is beneficial against anxiety and depression. Available over the counter in capsules. It can also be drunk as a tea.

Echinacea
North American Indians have traditionally used this plant as an overall tonic to strengthen both the mind and body and to maintain the immune system. Capsules are generally anti-infective and used for treating colds and flu. They also help rebuild the immune system, particularly in the pelvic region, and may be taken after yeast infections, such as candida and thrush, and following cystitis. It is also recommended for treating glandular fever. Taken as a tea, it improves the circulation and may help in treating bronchitis. A practitioner may prescribe a tincture for this. It has been used to help restore the immune system in cancer patients following chemotherapy, but is not recommended for self-help.

Evening primrose oil
Evening primrose oil is a popular supplement that contains the nutrient gamma linoleic acid (GLA), used by the body for the formation of prostaglandins. Similar to hormones, these play a part in the regulation of the blood, skin, and reproductive functions. The body makes its own GLA but not always very effectively. Evening primrose oil is helpful in treating many different conditions, including PMS, painful breasts, and arthritis. Atopic eczema is thought to be caused by a deficiency of linoleic acid in the body and evening primrose oil may be taken internally for this condition and also applied directly on the lesions. Evening primrose oil may also benefit brittle hair and nails. Some herbalists believe it may help coronary heart disease. Evening primrose oil is available in liquid and capsules. Use as directed.

Fennel
This is excellent for toning up a sluggish system and for stimulating the appetite. An infusion of fennel on its own or mixed with chamomile and hops helps constipation.

Flax (linseed)

This small brown seed contains nutrients vital to the body's life processes and well-being. It is rich in omega-3 fatty acids, important in the prevention of serious degenerative illnesses such as heart disease, cancer, arteriosclerosis, high blood pressure, immune disorders, allergies, depression, and certain kinds of mental illness. Grind the linseeds or crush them in a pestle with a mortar and add them to any meal you choose—from breakfast cereal to soup, salad, and stew. Three teaspoons of linseed swallowed with water once a day, at the same time each day but not at mealtimes, softens the consistency of bowel movements, alleviating the discomfort of hemorrhoids.

Ginger

This is the herb the Chinese use for treating morning sickness, motion sickness, indigestion, and nausea. Peel and grate the root to make an infusion of ginger tea for treating these digestive complaints or take one capsule up to three times daily. An infusion of ginger root is also helpful in treating most forms of arthritis and menstrual cramps, as well as helping raise the spirits of those suffering depression. Tablets are also effective for treating menstrual cramps: Take one up to three times a day. Ginger is said to stimulate the function of the lungs and a practitioner may prescribe a tincture for treating bronchitis. An infusion of ginger and spring onion is a traditional remedy for colds and flu.

Ginkgo biloba

This herb stimulates the blood supply to the brain. Older people with circulatory problems may benefit from one capsule a day. It may also help alleviate the symptoms of post-viral fatigue. It may help Alzheimer sufferers; it is thought to help memory loss. It has an antioxidant action and it is thought to protect cells and slow down the aging process. Use only over-the-counter preparations. Caution: some people cannot tolerate even small doses.

Ginseng

This is a wonderful tonic that stimulates and helps to restore the whole body, increases endurance, helps counter stress, and boosts energy. Overdosage of ginseng causes restlessness, irritability, muscular aches, and tension (particularly in the neck and shoulders). Ginseng is reputed to stimulate energy in all the body's organs and may be helpful in treating some forms of impotence and loss of libido in both men and women. However, ginseng can overenergize certain types of women and prolonged use or high doses should be avoided during pregnancy. Two cups of ginseng tea taken daily may help alleviate menopausal hot flashes. Ginseng should not be taken by those who are suffering from fever or flu symptoms or who have high blood pressure. Ginseng is available in many forms. Use as directed or consult your herbalist. If you are taking a vitamin C supplement, allow two hours between taking this and taking ginseng, as this vitamin can interfere with the body's ability to absorb ginseng.

Guarana

The seeds of this herb contain a small amount of caffeine, which is partly why it is so widely recognized as an energy booster. Researchers in a number of countries have found it to be effective in the treatment of Alzheimer's disease. It revitalizes mind and body and may be used as a pick-me-up in times of low energy.

Kombucha

This tonic has been brewed and drunk in China for more than 2,000 years and is claimed to have strengthening, rejuvenating, and revivifying properties. It is a heavy mixture of yeast and bacteria that contains a rich variety of B-complex vitamins, folic acid, a powerful detoxifying agent, glucuronic acid, an antibacterial, and usnic acid, an antiviral agent. These combine to help repair and strengthen the body's connective tissue. It is said to help prevent serious illness because of its immune-enhancing properties and to keep aging at bay, cure arthritis, and reduce the risk of cancer or the size of existing tumors.

Propolis

Propolis seems to stimulate the immune system to form antibodies that differentiate between useful and harmful bacteria. It is also helpful in the treatment of cystitis: Take one capsule or tablet three times a day, or as directed. An alternative medical practitioner may prescribe a course of propolis and pollen for the treatment of prostate problems. Women suffering from vulvitis (inflammation of the vulva) may be advised to take 3 g propolis a day for three days and then 2 g a day for eight days. Propolis is also available as a liquid: Drink 4 to 10 drops in half a glass of warm water once or twice a day.

Reishi mushroom

The reishi mushroom is considered an important energy tonic. It is claimed to stimulate the immune system and is officially listed in Japan as a substance for treating cancer. It can also be used for deficiency conditions and to fortify the body's natural vigor. Use capsules as directed.

Royal jelly

This tonic is the natural food of the queen bee, who is much bigger and lives 60 times longer than the other bees! The power of royal jelly has been well-known in China and other Eastern countries for many centuries. Even today the Chinese give injections of royal jelly to cure arthritis. Royal jelly is claimed to enhance the general level of well-being, to stimulate the immune system, and to increase stamina and energy levels. It has a natural diuretic action and also helps to relieve allergies and asthma, to heal wounds, and to purify the blood. Some researchers believe royal jelly boosts the body's ability to handle the side effects of chemotherapy and radiation in cancer treatment. To improve and maintain well-being, use capsules as directed on the package or by your herbalist. You can also take it as a liquid tonic in a single-dose vial for a fast-acting pick-me-up, but do not take a vial every day as you may get more energy than you need.

Saw palmetto

The saw palmetto berries are claimed to be an excellent energy and sex tonic, particularly for men experiencing impotence or prostate problems. The North American Indians have a long tradition of using the berries for catarrh and congestion of the lungs. Saw palmetto is also used to treat urinary problems. Caution: Do not substitute saw palmetto for medical treatment.

Chinese Herbs

For thousands of years the Chinese have been using herbs as medicinal preparations to build up the immune system, warm or cleanse the blood, balance and regulate the body's functions, and promote physical and mental well-being. Chinese herbal medicine is one of the oldest systems of medicine in the world and is part of traditional Chinese medicine, which also includes acupuncture and massage. Traditional Chinese medicine is a mixture of healing and philosophy in which the aim is to restore and maintain balance and harmony within the whole person. There is no place for the Western concept of simply treating a specific illness or disease; Chinese doctors take a holistic approach to their patients. Humans, like everything in the universe, are seen as being subject to the Great Principle—the laws of Yin and Yang. Energy, or chi, is divided into two complementary forms. Yin energy is female, soft, cold, dark, and wet, while Yang energy is male, hard, warm, bright, and dry. Good health and general well-being depend on a proper balance of Yin and Yang energy. Chinese practitioners believe that herbal medicine works by clearing the energy channels within the body and then restoring balance and normality. Any illness is thought to be caused by an imbalance of Yin and Yang within the body or a blockage of the circulation of chi.

The ingredients in Chinese herbal medicine include the seeds, roots, stems, sap, and twigs of plants, as well as the leaves, berries, and flowers. Chinese herbal medicine is rich in herbs that have been used over the centuries to maintain and enhance mental and physical well-being, as well as to address all kinds of complaints, such as chronic fatigue, stress, and loss of libido.

As we become more interested in alternative methods of healing, many of us are exploring the benefits of traditional Chinese herbal remedies. However, as with all potent remedies, Chinese herbal remedies should be treated with respect and caution. Always seek treatment and obtain remedies from a well-established, thoroughly trained practitioner who will prepare a prescription suited to your own individual needs; the remedies should not be administered to anyone else. Preparations bought from health food stores are safe to take provided you follow the dosage instructions very carefully. If you have an existing medical condition or are pregnant or breast-feeding, consult a conventional medical practitioner before self-administering these herbs.

Treating skin disorders with Chinese herbs

Chinese herbal medicine has caught the attention of many research establishments in the Western world as a result of its successful treatment of skin disorders, particularly serious eczema and acne.

Interest in herbal medicine is particularly high in Great Britain, where some studies have shown promising results. British dermatologists first became interested in traditional Chinese herbal medicine when they heard about a Chinese woman doctor working in London who had had significant success in treating skin complaints. Doctors at the Great Ormond Street Hospital in London conducted trials with children in 1990. They had such positive results that they extended the research to adults. They monitored the children and adults closely for any signs of side effects; the herbs were not found to be toxic or damaging to the liver when taken properly. The herbal mix they used for skin complaints had an anti-inflammatory, anti-itching, sedative effect on the skin and "cooled" the inflamed areas.

In the early 1990s, another trial was carried out at The Royal Free Hospital in London. Chinese herbs were used to treat chronic eczema and other severe skin conditions in 31 adults. The herbs were grown in mainland China and had been used for treating skin conditions there for several thousand years. The results of the trials in London were published in the medical journal *The Lancet* in 1992. All the patients who completed the study showed a marked improvement. Many of them felt they had been transformed by having a clear skin, free of irritation and inflammation, for the first time in their lives. Most of the people in the trial had tried several conventional treatments without success.

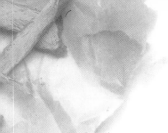

Chinese herbs

Astragalus (huang chi)

This is a great immune enhancer, boosting the production of white and red blood cells, interferon, immunoglobulins, and the function of the adrenal cortex. It is being investigated in this country for use with cancer and AIDS patients. An excellent tonic when associated with dong quai, it is considered an energizer for those who are physically active. It is a Yang tonic, widely available from health food stores. Do not take if you are feverish or if you are undergoing chemotherapy.

Codonopsis root (dang shen)

Thought of as milder and softer than ginseng, this herb is used as an energy booster and tonic for improving general well-being. It is as famous as ginseng in China, where it is also used to strengthen the lungs, spleen, and stomach. It is good for promoting the appetite and can be used to treat heartburn. It can be given to children more safely than ginseng. It is sold in Asian markets and may be taken with astragalus or angelica.

Dong quai (Chinese angelica root)

This herb is called the women's ginseng and may benefit women with low sex drives or those with gynecological problems such as PMS, menstrual cramps, and hot flashes. It is as widely consumed as ginseng and ginger, a popular male tonic combination. Dong quai is a blood tonic, rich in vitamins and minerals, and is thought to help prevent anemia and reduce high blood pressure. It is also helpful in treating exhaustion and debility. *Note:* Do not use Dong quai during pregnancy, if you are planning pregnancy, or during a period if the flow is unusually heavy.

Fang feng

This herbal remedy is thought to boost the body's natural immunity and may be beneficial to convalescents. It is also used to treat muscular spasms. Fang feng is available from most Asian markets and Chinese herbalists.

Ginseng

Ren shen is the Chinese ginseng, useful for toning up a system weakened by disease, overwork, or old age. It is both a stimulant and a sedative, according to the body's needs, and very useful in combating the effects of stress. San qi, or tian qi, is another form of ginseng that has been shown to give pain relief, lower blood pressure and cholesterol levels, and to reduce swelling. Xi yang shen is American ginseng, a mild and gentle tonic. Ginseng is probably the most celebrated herbal aphrodisiac and has long been revered in the East for its recuperative and revitalizing powers. It is so powerful it may be too strong for women, who can easily overdose on ginseng, becoming more aggressive and irritable. For this reason it is best prescribed by a traditional Chinese medicine practitioner, although most practitioners believe that Chinese angelica root is a better tonic for the majority of women.

Gou qi zi (Fructus Lycii)

This is a Yin tonic and a gentle toner for the kidneys and liver. It also helps poor eyesight and even benefits the complexion. Modern research shows that the fruit promotes regeneration of liver cells and lowers blood cholesterol levels. It can also prevent atherosclerosis. It is traditionally believed to lengthen life and create a feeling of general well-being. It is available from most Chinese herbalists. If you find it difficult to digest, it can be taken with ginger.

He shou wu

This rejuvenating tonic is thought to prolong youth, promote vigor, and prevent prematurely gray hair. It is used to help with infertility problems in both sexes and is also thought to strengthen the heart and to lower blood pressure. It is widely available in health food stores and from herbalists.

Licorice (gan cao)

Used by the Chinese for over 5,000 years, this remarkable root helps combat the ill effects of drugs, balances the body's blood sugar levels, and relieves pain and spasms in the digestive system. It is considered a particularly effective herb for treating poor digestion, although it should not be used as a laxative. Licorice is used in combination for treating coughs and sore throats and for healing sores.

Rehmannia (shu di huang)

This is a good herbal remedy for counteracting fatigue and promoting general healing. It is used to treat anemia and is thought to speed the healing of injured bones. It is available from most Chinese herbalists.

Schisandra (wu wei zi)

This is a famous herb, used as a sex booster and highly valued by Chinese women. It also softens and beautifies the skin and is thought to preserve youth and beauty. It balances the nervous system, increases endurance, and reduces fatigue. It can help lower blood pressure, reduce hot flashes or excessive sweating, and improve night vision. It is easily available in health food stores and from herbalists.

Warning

Traditional Chinese herbs are very powerful and should not be taken without expert advice. In the wrong dosages and with inexpert diagnosis they can be harmful. Taking various combinations of these herbs is also potentially dangerous. Always seek a qualified practitioner's advice.

Some reports have associated the use of Chinese herbs for eczema with liver failure. This can be avoided by visiting a reputable practitioner, who will make up a formula for your unique requirements. Pregnant women should not take herbal tonics without seeking the advice of a qualified practitioner. Even ginseng root and ginger may be too much of a stimulant for a certain mind-body type and could be dangerous for those with high blood pressure.

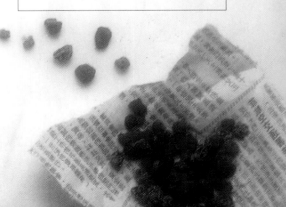

Flower Remedies and Tissue Salts

Bach flower remedies are designed to relieve negative feelings, such as pessimism, apprehension, and resentment, while biochemic tissue salts aim to help restore the balance of inorganic minerals in the body.

The Bach remedies are infusions of flowers that are preserved in alcohol. During the 1930s their discoverer, British bacteriologist and homeopath Edward Bach, reached the conclusion that a patient's mental and emotional state can affect the body's ability to heal. It is only comparatively recently that conventional medical science has acknowledged the importance of mental attitude as well as physical condition in the healing process. Edward Bach's approach was holistic: he believed that a physician should "treat the patient and not the disease," and his research led him to conclude that negative thinking is at the root of most physical and emotional problems.

Closely attuned to nature and deeply sensitive to the energies and qualities of plants, Bach developed 38 remedies as a complete system of treatment for all negative states of mind, rather than cures for specific illnesses. Seven basic negative emotional states have been identified: fear, uncertainty, insufficient interest in the present, loneliness, oversensitivity, despondency or despair, and overconcern for the welfare of others. All but one of the remedies are derived from flowers. Rock water remedy is taken from natural springs or wells that have a long history of healing. An additional remedy—the rescue remedy—is a combination of five others (cherry plum, clematis, impatiens, rock rose, and star of Bethlehem) and is designed to provide emergency relief in times of severe stress or shock.

Up to six negative conditions may be treated at the same time. It is essential to be both searching and completely truthful with yourself when analyzing your state of mind. Once you have recognized the underlying emotional condition that is causing distress or illness, you can treat it with the appropriate remedy. One treatment bottle lasts about three weeks. Trained Bach counselors can advise and assist with this process.

The 38 remedies

Fear
Aspen, cherry plum, mimulus, red chestnut, rock rose.
Uncertainty
Cerato, gentian, gorse, hornbeam, scleranthus, wild oat.
Insufficent interest in the present
Chestnut bud, clematis, honeysuckle, mustard, olive, white chestnut, wild rose.
Loneliness
Heather, impatiens, water violet.
Oversensitivity
Agrimony, centaury, holly, walnut.
Despondency or despair
Crab apple, elm, larch, oak, pine, star of Bethlehem, sweet chestnut, willow.
Overconcern for welfare of others
Chicory, beech, rock water, vervain, vine.

Making the remedies

Bach flower remedies are still made at The Bach Center, located at Bach's house–Mount Vernon–in Wallingford, England, following the original method. Only perfect flowers are used, and immediately after picking they are placed in glass bowls of spring water and left for three hours in full sun. This is thought to imprint the essence of the flower on the water and is known as potentizing. The potentized water is then mixed with an equal quantity of brandy to preserve it before bottling. This produces the stock bottles.

Ready-made treatment bottles, which are fitted with a dispensing dropper, are available and stock bottles may be bought at many health food stores. You can prepare your own treatment bottle, using a single remedy or a mixture, depending on the negative feelings you wish to alleviate. Mix two drops of each required stock bottle remedy with one ounce of pure spring water in a bottle with a dispensing dropper. Always store in a cool place. To use them, either place three to four drops directly on the tongue or mix a few drops with water and drink it, four times a day. Do not touch the liquid with your fingers. The Bach Center emphasizes that, while Bach flower remedies are completely safe, they should not be regarded as a substitute for conventional medical treatment.

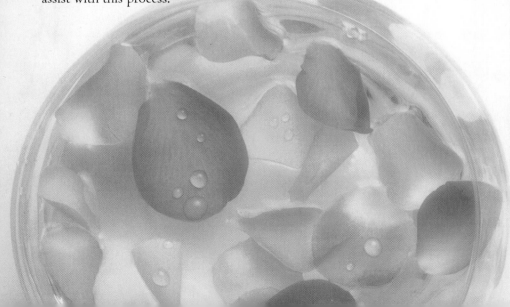

Tissue Salts

Also known as biochemic remedies, tissue salts are designed to restore an imbalance of inorganic minerals in the body. They were developed in the 19th century by a German homeopathic physician, Wilhelm Schuessler, who believed that a deficiency or imbalance of mineral salts in the cells of the body was the cause of illness and disease. Twelve basic tissue salts, each with very specific properties, are thought to be essential for healing and well-being. It is important to understand how the salts interrelate, as well as how they work individually. Practitioners may prescribe a number of different tissue salts to be taken in a specific order to treat certain conditions. They are also a popular form of self-help, and advocates recommend using them for various minor conditions, such as pimples, cramps, and headaches.

Like homeopathic remedies, tissue salts are prepared in minute, very dilute quantities. They are taken in tablet form and placed directly on the tongue, where assimilation is thought to begin immediately. They may be taken every 30 minutes for treating acute conditions and every two to three hours for more prolonged illnesses.

The 12 tissue salts and their uses

Biochemic No. and Name	Chemical Name	Function	Conditions Treated
1. Calc. Fluor.	Calcium fluoride	Gives elasticity to tissues	Hemorrhoids, varicose veins, muscular weakness, poor circulation
2. Calc. Phos.	Calcium phosphate	Bone and teeth formation	Chilblains, indigestion of food, lowered vitality during convalescence
3. Calc. Sulf.	Calcium sulfate	Blood purifier	Spots, pimples, slow-healing wounds
4. Ferr. Phos.	Iron phosphate	Constituent of oxygen-carrying red blood cells	Skin inflammation, fever, sore throat, muscular rheumatism. Internally, to treat the common cold; externally, for cuts and abrasions
5. Kali. Mur.	Potassium chloride	Balances watery emissions	Congested conditions, particularly whitish catarrhal discharges
6. Kali. Phos.	Potassium phosphate	Nerve nutrient	Nervous tension, depression; loss of sleep, irritability, nervous headaches, general debility
7. Kali. Sulf.	Potassium sulfate	Promotes and maintains healthy skin	Yellowish exudations and discharges of the skin, nose, or throat; brittle nails, poor condition of hair and scalp
8. Mag. Phos.	Magnesium phosphate	Nutrient for nerve and muscle fiber	Darting pains, cramps, hiccups, colic
9. Nat. Mur.	Sodium chloride	Controls the body's water distribution	Watery colds and runny nose
10. Nat. Phos.	Sodium phosphate	Acid-alkaline cell regulator	Acidity, heartburn, indigestion
11. Nat. Sulf.	Sodium sulfate	Body water balancer	Bilious conditions, colic, headaches
12. Silica	Silica, Silicon dioxide, Silicic acid	Elimination of toxic accumulations and waste material	Pus formations, boils, sties

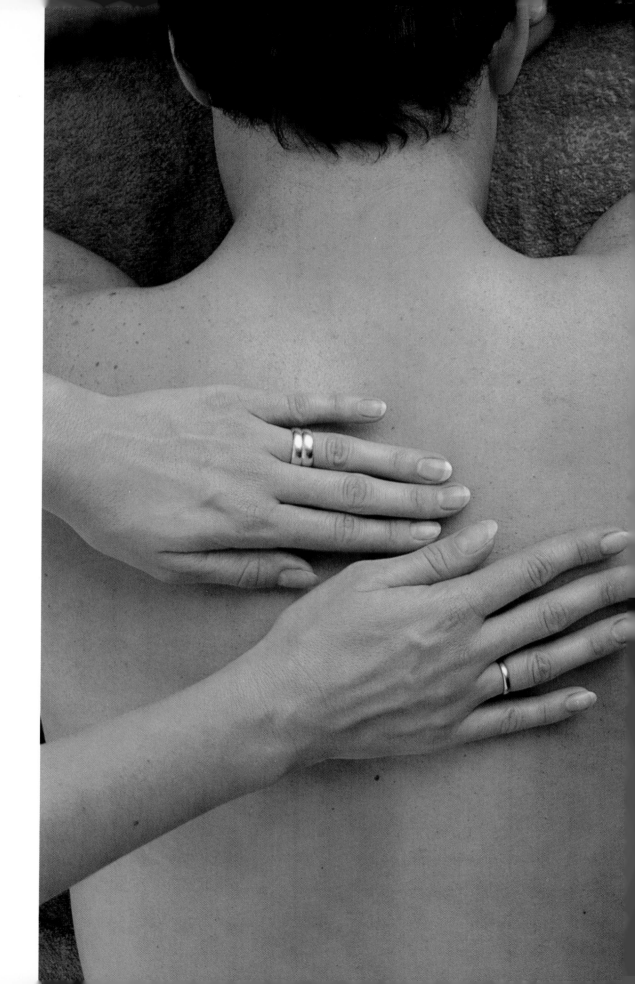

4
Practicing Prevention

It is easier to prevent serious illness than cure it. By focusing on prevention we can maximize our potential for good health and well-being. We are lucky that there are now so many natural, alternative therapies that enable us to participate fully in creating our own personal preventive healthcare program.

Many of the natural therapies available help to reduce the negative effects of the ever-increasing amount of stress we have in our lives and promote a greater sense of well-being for both mind and body.

For some, massage will provide the answer, while for others, it might be a dose of flower remedies or acupuncture. In this chapter we explore some of the alternative therapies that can help keep our bodies well in a nonintrusive, natural way.

Vaccination and Immunization

The artificial stimulation of immunity against certain infectious diseases has been one of the outstanding success stories of this century. With the introduction of mass immunization programs in the 1940s and 1950s, former childhood killers like diphtheria and polio have all but disappeared, and smallpox has been eradicated. There has also been a dramatic decline in the incidence of measles, mumps, and rubella (German measles) since the introduction of the MMR vaccine.

Immunization is important not just to protect individuals, but to keep disease levels low in the community. When immunization rates fall, outbreaks occur. Immunization has been so successful that most of us have no memory of the devastation caused by epidemics of childhood illnesses. The danger is that people may become lax and that crippling diseases like polio and diphtheria could return. The alternative view on immunization is that it weakens the body's natural ability to fight infection. But state and local authorities require immunizations before a child enters school, so discuss the matter with your pediatrician before deciding against inoculations for your child.

Recommended schedule

Hepatitis B
Given at birth; at 2 mos.; and between 6 and 18 mos.

Diphtheria, Tetanus, Pertussis (DTP)
Given at 2, 4, and 6 mos.; then between 12 and 18 mos.; and between 4 and 6 yrs. (alternately, DTAP is given at these times). Between 11 and 16 yrs., DT boosters are given.

Hemophilus influenza B
Given between 2 and 4 mos.; then between 12 and 15 mos.

Polio
Given between 2 and 4 mos.; then between 6 and 18 mos.; and between 4 and 6 yrs.

Measles, Mumps, Rubella (MMR)
Given between 12 and 15 mos.; and between 4 and 6 yrs.

Chickenpox
Given between 12 and 18 mos.

Most vaccinations and immunizations are done in early childhood, with boosters given in adolescence.

Types of immunization

Most immunizations are given by injection into the arm or buttock. Some, like the polio vaccine, are given by mouth. Immunization can be either active or passive. The most common type is active immunization (also known as vaccination). The vaccine contains specially treated microorganisms that trigger the body's immune system to produce antibodies without giving a full-blown illness. The immune system then retains a "memory" of the disease and if the person is exposed to it in the future he or she produces antibodies to fight off infection. In passive immunization, antibodies to a disease are injected into the bloodstream providing immediate, though short-term, protection.

Vaccines known as live vaccines are prepared from viruses and bacteria that have lost their virulence but still provoke antibody formation. They include the yellow fever, oral polio, and BCG (against TB) vaccines. Most of the other vaccines are made from dead microorganisms that have been killed in such a way as to preserve their ability to confer immunity.

Adverse reactions

Modern vaccines cause few if any side effects and these are likely to be mild. The most usual are soreness, redness, and swelling at the site of the injection, a flulike feeling, and/or headache. Babies may be fretful and slightly feverish. Rest, plenty of fluids, and a painkiller usually ease these minor symptoms. Very occasionally immunization may provoke a severe reaction such as a seizure.

Whooping cough
The whooping cough part of the triple vaccine–diphtheria, tetanus, and pertussis (whooping cough)–has been the subject of a lot of controversy. In some extremely rare instances it has been suggested that it could provoke a reaction that may lead to permanent brain damage. So far studies have failed to find a convincing link between the vaccine and permanent brain damage and all the evidence suggests that the dangers to a young baby or child of getting the disease far outweigh any risk from the vaccine.

Childhood immunization
Infants and children should be immunized against diphtheria, tetanus, pertussis, (whooping cough), polio, measles, mumps, and rubella (German measles), and a type of meningitis called Hemophilus influenza (Hib). Immunization for hepatitis B and chickenpox is also advisable (schedule, page 68).

Travel immunization
Travelers to destinations in parts of the Third World are recommended to have certain immunizations, although only yellow fever is likely to be compulsory for certain areas. These include booster shots of diphtheria, tetanus, and polio and other vaccines such as typhoid, hepatitis A and B, rabies, and meningitis. If you are intending to travel to such destinations, check which immunizations are required a few months before departure.

Flu immunization
People who are weakened by other illnesses, those with certain chronic health problems, and some older people may find it harder to fight off flu and may benefit from being immunized.

Alternatives to vaccination

Despite the success of mass immunization campaigns in combating infectious diseases, vaccination remains a point of contention between conventional doctors, most of whom are in favor of it, and some alternative practitioners, who may be against it.

According to the viewpoint against vaccinations, they pose an unnecessary stress on the immune system by filling the body with toxins that cause the immune system to overreact, creating a gross imbalance in the body's natural harmony. Some alternative practitioners argue that healthy individuals possess strong natural defenses against illness that protect against disease, making vaccination unnecessary. If we do fall ill, it is always for a reason– usually because the vital force or energy that each of us possesses is lowered or out of balance. This view holds that any imbalance in vital energy is best corrected by the use of herbal or homeopathic remedies tailored to the individual and designed to strengthen the immune system. However, those whose innate resistance is lowered may be advised to have conventional vaccination.

Some homeopathic practitioners go still further, claiming that vaccination actively damages the immune system. In the short term they claim this damage can make children more susceptible to problems such as middle-ear infection, sore throats, coughs, colds, and chest infections. In the long term they blame vaccination for the increase in serious problems such as autoimmune diseases (in which the body turns against itself), multiple sclerosis, asthma and other allergies, behavioral problems, and even AIDS. These people believe that only children who are constitutionally susceptible to the infectious illnesses against which children are immunized will contract them, and that they are only dangerous to those whose vital force is weakened, either because of their constitutional makeup or because of conventional methods of treatment such as antibiotics. Many homeopaths argue that rather than being vaccinated, children should be treated with remedies designed to strengthen their individual constitutions (constitutional remedies) and build up their natural defense mechanisms so that their bodies are able to combat infection.

Homeopathy

Homeopathy uses highly diluted, minute quantities of natural substances to aid the body's own process of recovery. It is based on the theory that "like cures like," in other words, a substance that causes the same symptoms as a disease will also be able to treat it. The name homeopathy comes from "homeo," or "similar," and "pathy," meaning "disease."

Homeopaths believe that the more the remedy is diluted, the more effective it is. The most commonly available homeopathic remedies are usually diluted to 1/1,000,000 of the strength of the original active substance. This strength is described as 6x on the label. However, practitioners often prescribe remedies of 30x and may even prescribe some as dilute as 10m (a 10,000-fold dilution). These numbers and letters refer to the homeopathic potency: The higher the number, the more dilute and the more effective the substance is thought to be. This principle of dilution is the one that has caused the greatest controversy about homeopathy in conventional medical circles.

The next important principle of homeopathy is that the practitioner must treat the whole person, not simply the symptoms of illness. Homeopaths take a holistic approach, believing that all the symptoms, and the patient's character and lifestyle must be assessed before a remedy can be prescribed. These are thought to be closely interconnected and their relationships and patterns must be traced. A homeopathic doctor may ask questions that might seem quite extraordinary and unlike anything conventional healthcare professionals ask. At the initial consultation, time is taken obtaining a full holistic diagnosis of the patient's symptoms, lifestyle, and medical history.

A homeopath will often prescribe completely different remedies for two patients suffering from the same disease because of this holistic approach. In addition, he or she will prescribe with very precise details of the symptoms in mind. For example, a patient who feels nauseated after eating will probably respond to a different remedy from one who feels sick when hungry.

The final principle of homeopathy has also raised controversy. The healing process is thought to start inside the body and work toward the outside, with symptoms moving in the same direction. Consequently, as one internal symptom improves, another external symptom may develop. This may mean that a patient feels worse before feeling better.

Modern science remains divided on the subject, but both people and animals have responded positively to homeopathic treatment. It is unquestionably a gentle approach to helping the body maintain and restore health and balance, and it is especially suited to the elderly, the very young, and those with allergies. It is completely safe, nontoxic, and free of serious side effects.

Samuel Hahnemann

Although some of the theories and practices of homeopathy were known to the fifth-century Greek physician Hippocrates and were widely used for centuries in Ayurvedic medicine in India, the 18th-century German doctor Samuel Hahnemann is regarded as the father of the modern therapy.

Hahnemann realized that quinine, used to treat malaria, produced similar symptoms to the disease: chills and sweating. Having read of the theory that "like cures like" in W. Cullen's *Materia Medica*, Hahnemann began to experiment on himself, systematically testing many substances–in high doses–and keeping careful notes of the symptoms they produced. He then applied this so-called law of similars to his patients, treating them with diluted doses and achieving great success.

Hahnemann went on to develop his theory that the more dilute the remedy, the more potent it was.

The Western world's disillusionment with conventional medical treatment has led to the increased popularity of homeopathic remedies during this century.

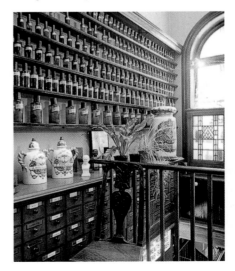

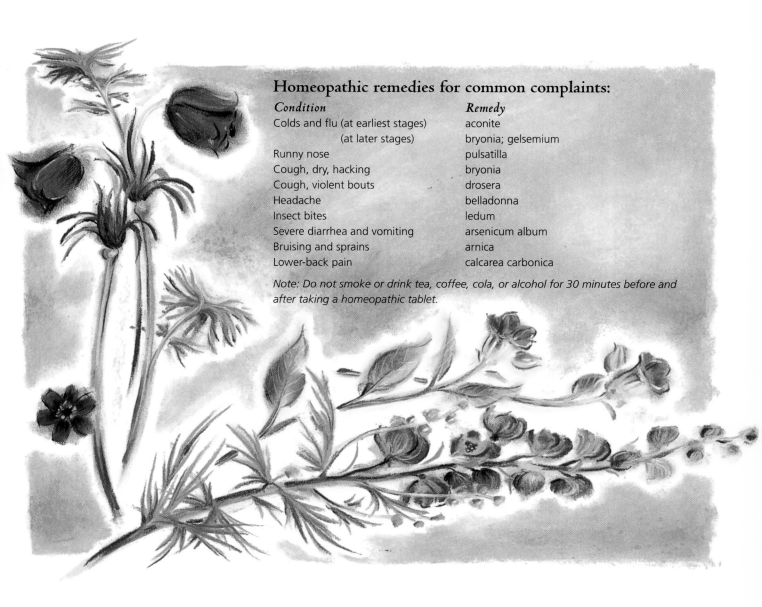

Homeopathic remedies for common complaints:

Condition	Remedy
Colds and flu (at earliest stages)	aconite
(at later stages)	bryonia; gelsemium
Runny nose	pulsatilla
Cough, dry, hacking	bryonia
Cough, violent bouts	drosera
Headache	belladonna
Insect bites	ledum
Severe diarrhea and vomiting	arsenicum album
Bruising and sprains	arnica
Lower-back pain	calcarea carbonica

Note: Do not smoke or drink tea, coffee, cola, or alcohol for 30 minutes before and after taking a homeopathic tablet.

Preventive homeopathy

Samuel Hahnemann believed strongly that a healthy body was better able to fight off illness. For this reason, he placed strong emphasis on preventing ill-health. Hahnemann was also one of the earliest doctors to stress the vital importance of good public hygiene, as well as good food and a healthy lifestyle, to aid in the prevention of disease.

Although there is a wide variety of homeopathic remedies to help in the prevention of colds, flu, whooping cough, and other infectious diseases, homeopathic practitioners also stress the importance of receiving prompt treatment for minor ills to help prevent the development of more serious complications. For example, the early control of diarrhea and vomiting avoids dehydration and protracted illness; arnica following injury reduces or prevents bruising, blood loss, and wound infection and promotes healing, enabling the sufferer to avoid serious secondary conditions and shortening convalescence. The prompt treatment of colds and flu can prevent secondary chest infections—important for the healthy but essential for those with asthma or emphysema.

In addition, homeopaths believe that treating future parents can reduce chronic illness in their children.

Massage

The benefits of massage cannot be overstated. Massage helps to bring about balance between body, mind, and spirit and encourages the body's own healing processes while assisting in clearing the mind of stress, hectic thought processes, and tension. It is a chance to let the mind go and to tune in to our bodies.

Massage has seen a resurgence in popularity in the West, particularly in the last decade. It was once confined to the gym for the exclusive benefit of athletes and sports people, a luxury enjoyed only by the wealthy, or those enjoying the dubious benefits of the seedier side of life. The rise in its popularity serves as evidence of the growing needs of individuals to seek pleasure and health—enhancing forms of relaxation as a means to combat the stresses brought on us all by our daily lives.

Massage aims to induce relaxation of both mind and body, but it can also be used to alleviate disorders of the body. Circulation can be improved and therapeutic massage may be used to help treat heart disorders, back pain, blood pressure, sleeping disorders, and various joint and muscle problems.

Eastern forms of massage have found their way to the West with increasing strength during the last decade. There are as many forms of massage as there are cultures, each with its own unique flavor.

Making the most of massage

There are many forms of massage available and this can seem confusing at first. It is a good idea to consider what you seek to gain from regular treatment when making your choice.

In order to gain the greatest benefit from your treatments it is important that you are able to let go fully during the session and place implicit trust in the practitioner. The environment in which you receive your treatment is important, too. A room that is clean, warm, and softly lit will add to the process. The practitioner may offer relaxation music. Gentle, soothing color schemes and soft furnishings with homey touches will enhance your session.

The massage couch or table should be sturdy, supportive, and comfortable. Cushions or padding may be offered to support your spine if you suffer from pain in the lower back. Fresh towels and covers should always be used for each client. If the practitioner works on the floor, an exercise mat or mattress may be used. Again, removable covers or towels should be used and they should be clean.

The practitioner will do her best to help you to relax prior to working on your body. He or she may ask a few general medical questions, ask you how you are feeling right now, or you may need to fill in a detailed medical history questionnaire. You will be engaged in discussion about your requirements, which will help you to develop a rapport with the practitioner.

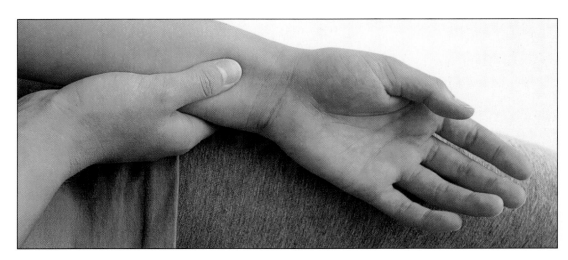

Asthma acupressure
Place your thumb on your wrist below the wrist crease and between the two tendons. Press firmly and make small circular movements. Pressing this point can help reduce and relieve an asthma attack, nausea, morning sickness, anxiety, and fatigue.

Choosing a massage therapy

Massage can be broken down into several types, which are detailed below. It is wise to bear in mind that massage is a universal art and influences from many cultures can be seen in holistic massage, while other forms remain quite specific and true to their origin and tradition.

Holistic massage

This is a term used to denote treatment of the person as a whole–that is, all aspects of your being will be taken into account, such as whether or not you display symptoms of a disorder, have an injury, or are depressed. Holistic massage is usually a full-body massage using a light vegetable oil base. The oil contains valuable nutrients and vitamins that travel into the body's systems through the layers of dermis after application. A full-body massage will normally follow a specific route, generally commencing with the back, back of legs, head, neck and shoulders, arms and hands, torso, abdomen, front of legs and feet, although this may be altered to suit the client's needs.

Those trained in holistic massage will use a variety of techniques and draw from a range of movements to provide the most effective treatment for the client. Holistic massage will not follow a rigidly structured pattern as used in Swedish massage or aromatherapy massage, for example. It will involve many long, connective strokes and the practitioner will strive to remain in physical contact with the client throughout the treatment. It may be appropriate to use deep pressure on one client, or very gentle pressure on another. This the practitioner will gauge by placing his or her hands on the body, receiving information through the hands and working accordingly. Holistic massage is very soothing, relaxing, and stress relieving.

Swedish massage

This is the type most often used in gyms but has regained popularity in general practice during the last decade. Often talcum powder will be used instead of oil as this allows a firmer grip between hand and skin. The massage generally follows a routine and can be used in a curative manner for disorders ranging from tennis elbow to stiffness in the neck. Machines such as G5 (vibrating pads that are placed on fleshy parts of the body such as thighs or buttocks) will be used to improve local circulation and muscle tone.

Swedish massage is good for those who require a firmer form of massage and those who exercise vigorously. Massaging muscle groups prior to exercise can be beneficial, although some hours should pass between treatment and exercise. Conversely, massage immediately after exercise should be avoided, allowing time for the heart rate to settle and the body to return to its normal rhythm.

Aromatherapy massage

As well as the light flowing movements of lymphatic drainage, aromatherapy incorporates some of the firm Swedish massage techniques to release muscular tension; neuromuscular pressure techniques to reach deeply held tension in connective tissues; and Shiatsu pressures to release and harmonize the body's vital energy. One of the main aims of this massage technique is to introduce the essential oils into the recipient's body via the capillaries. Again, as in Swedish and holistic massage, a basic regimen will be followed, starting with the back.

A more detailed medical history may be taken, which sometimes includes a reflexology diagnosis on the feet, to determine particular physical problems, and a discussion about any current or past emotional problems. The oils used will be chosen in a holistic fashion with the aim of bringing about a balance between mind, body, and spirit.

Aromatherapy massage is notably very soothing and relaxing and a great stress reliever. Aromatherapy can also be used in other ways, by inhalation and bathing, for example.

Shiatsu

Shiatsu is a Japanese massage therapy that is growing steadily in popularity in the Western world. The word "shiatsu" means "finger pressure" in Japanese and used to be practiced almost entirely with the balls of the thumbs, which apply pressure to any or all of the hundreds of points located along the meridians (energy pathways) for several seconds at a time.

Shiatsu is a form of acupuncture without the needles, stimulating or relaxing the

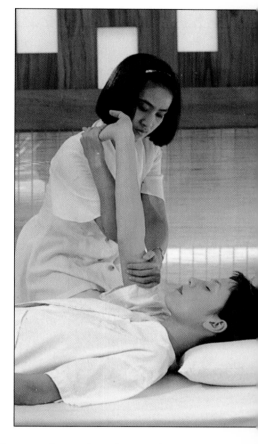

Shiatsu is a Japanese form of massage that focuses on precise pressure points on the body to promote well-being. Pressure is applied with the thumbs, fingertips, and even the elbows.

acupuncture points with the fingertips and even the elbows. There is also a general stroking over parts of the body to stimulate a harmonious flow of energy throughout the body.

Sometimes the practitioner uses gentle manipulation to stretch the meridians and to loosen joints. This helps tone up the body's energy, releasing lots of stress and tension, helping to alleviate symptoms of disorder, and preventing various unhealthy conditions.

Shiatsu is effective in treating the following conditions:
● asthma ● insomnia ● back and neck pain ● headache ● low vitality ● chronic fatigue ● digestive problems ● PMS
● menstrual cramps.

Do-In

Do-In is an ancient Chinese system of exercise that claims to help prevent illness and disease with a set of simple exercises that stimulate the meridians (also called energy channels or pathways). These meridians are linked to all the organs in the body and the exercises act as a form of self-massage, balancing the energy flow to the organs to help keep them healthy and toned. Do-In exercises were created to make the organs stronger, helping to prevent all sorts of health problems from heart and lung disease to arthritis, irritable bowel syndrome, and stress.

You can perform these exercises any time of day, but as with all forms of exercise, do not practice Do-In immediately after a meal. Wear comfortable, unrestricted clothing. If you do not have experience in Eastern movement systems it is probably a good idea to seek some instruction in the basics with a qualified, experienced teacher to confirm the accuracy of your positions. Since Do-In is related to Shiatsu, you should be able to find a teacher to instruct you on the positions of the meridians through a local Shiatsu practitioner or school.

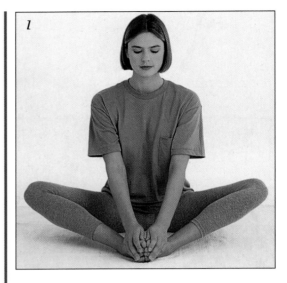

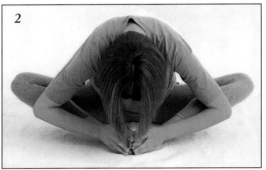

Heart-small intestine meridian
1. Sit with a straight, firm back, with your shoulders down and your legs open. The soles of your feet should be touching. Hold your feet around the toes and take a deep breath.
2. Slowly bend forward from your hips, exhaling as you bring your forehead down toward your feet and hands. Hold on a full breath cycle (one inhalation and one exhalation) and then slowly sit up as you inhale. Repeat at least twice.

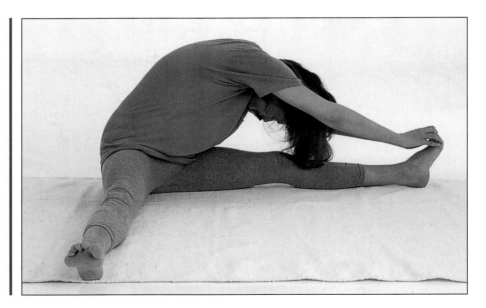

Liver-gall bladder meridian
Sit up straight and spread your legs as far apart as you can without straining. Inhale deeply and slowly. As you exhale, bend from the hip, stretching your arms over your left leg as you try to grasp your left foot. Do not raise your right buttock off the floor. Hold this position for two deep breaths and then repeat the exercise on the right side. Repeat at least twice.

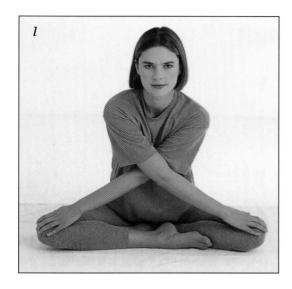

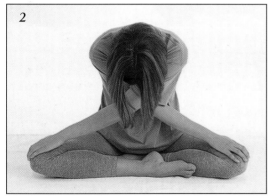

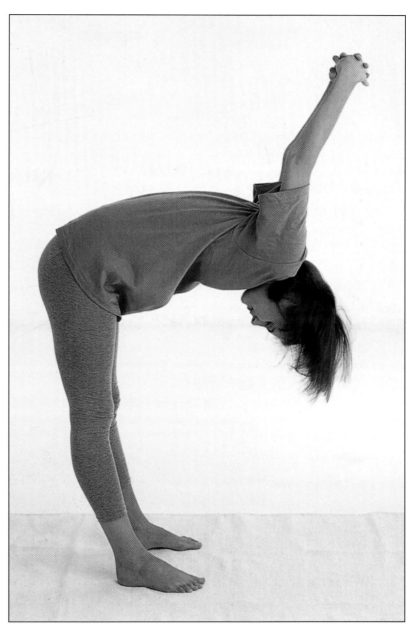

Circulation-pericardium meridian

1. Sit on the floor with your legs crossed, inhale and cross your arms and hold your knees.
2. As you exhale, slowly bend forward and gently try to press your knees to the floor. Alternate by crossing your legs and arms the other way and then repeat the process. Repeat at least twice.

Lung-large intestine meridian

Stand straight, firm, and centered, with your feet parallel and a shoulder-width apart. With your arms behind your back, hold your hands and lock your thumbs. Inhale deeply and slowly while you stretch your arms up behind you and slowly rise. Exhale and bend forward. Hold for a complete breath cycle. Repeat twice.

Aromatherapy

Aromatherapy is an ancient healing art that was practiced thousands of years ago in many cultures, including ancient Egypt, China, Persia, Greece, and Rome, when flowers were pressed to make healing remedies and natural medicines.

The modern revival of interest in aromatherapy came at the beginning of the 20th century, when many natural healing techniques enjoyed a renaissance. At this time, French chemist René Gattefosse, who was aware of the potency of the essential oils of plants, staged an experiment to prove their powers to the scientific community. Having badly burned his hand in his laboratory, he applied lavender oil to the burns on one part of his hand and treated the remaining burns in the conventional way. Witnesses were amazed to see that the part treated with lavender oil healed considerably faster than the rest and did not blister or scar. Thus began the modern rediscovery of the power of essential oils that can help prevent and treat all kinds of conditions, from minor skin rashes to serious illness.

Aromatherapy evolved through an understanding of the power of smell. When smells are inhaled they act on the sensitive olfactory nerves in the nose and rapidly transmit the message to the brain, and from there to other parts of the body. Each essential oil has a different smell and a wide variety of therapeutic properties. Aromatherapy can be used at home *(pages 78-79)* either in the bath or with a device that diffuses the aroma throughout the room. It is increasingly used in combination with massage. The way this is practiced today is a combination of using essential oils—the heavily scented, potent extracts of plants that contain the smell "essence" of that plant—and applying them to the body, using soft- and deep-tissue massage techniques that can be either relaxing or stimulating, depending on your needs and condition. When essential oils are used with massage, small quantities of the essence are absorbed through the skin and its healing effect travels straight to the nervous system.

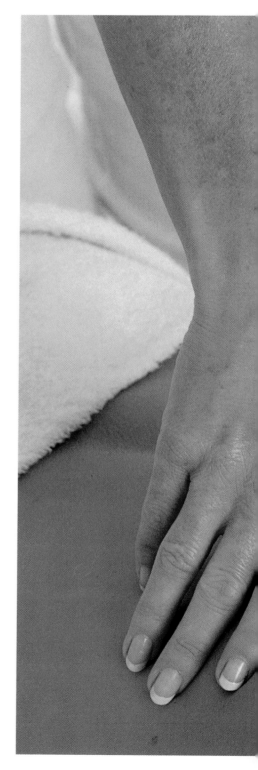

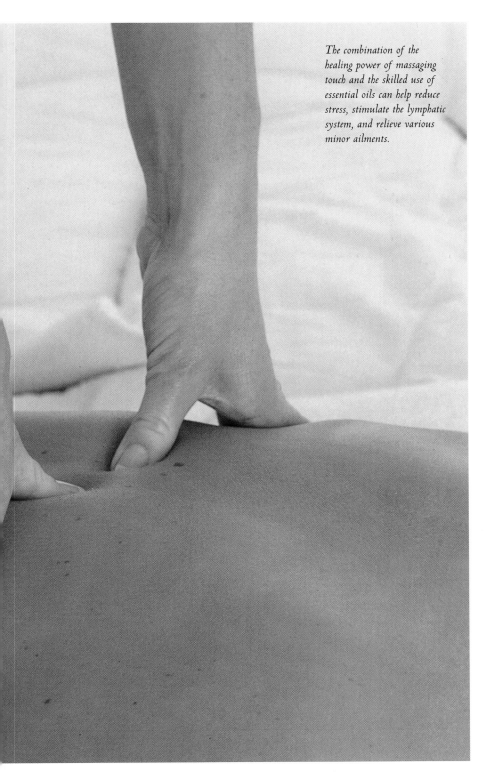

The combination of the healing power of massaging touch and the skilled use of essential oils can help reduce stress, stimulate the lymphatic system, and relieve various minor ailments.

Massage aromatherapy

It is important to choose a massage therapist who uses aromatherapy carefully as this technique has become very popular and many therapists are practicing at beauty salons and health spas without having undergone the thorough training that is essential for the safe use of such potent oils. Always choose a massage therapist who is state-licensed.

Proper massage training requires a detailed study of anatomy and physiology. A practitioner is expected to possess knowledge of common disorders and illnesses ranging from skin complaints and stress-related mental conditions to physical problems such as muscle fatigue or joint disorders. However, such a therapist is not expected to have the knowledge of a doctor, although much focus is placed on the correct "diagnosis" of conditions since the oils used in treatment will act directly on the muscles and organs of the body.

Case histories and subsequent assessment are pivotal to the training. The therapist has to find out the medical history of the client, determine what the client wishes to have treated, and then decide on the appropriate oils. A trainee is required to spend many hours studying case histories and attending supervised sessions.

The aromatherapy massage technique will assist in draining the lymph system. This helps the body expel accumulated toxins, or stress crystals, that build up in the body's tissues. The technique used is gentle, soothing, and relaxing. The aim is to promote the introduction of the oils into the client's bloodstream and thereby to the relevant organs needing attention. The technique may also incorporate a study of a range of acupressure points to enhance the draining process and the ingestion of oil.

Aromatherapists in some countries must learn the chemical constituents of 40 to 50 commonly used oils and their beneficial effects. They also have to know how to mix a variety of oils and are expected to understand the importance of correct blending in treatment.

Essential oils in the home

Aromatherapy has many practical applications in the home. As well as using the oils for relaxing baths and massage, we can scent our environment to promote auras of happiness, calm, and relaxation. We can use aromatherapy to cure minor ailments and injuries, and since certain oils have antiseptic properties, they are good for the sickroom; others can be used as disinfectants or insect sprays.

There are a few things to remember when using essential oils at home. Always read the labels and instructions for the oil. Look for essential oils that contain as much original purity as possible. Pure, undiluted essential oils should never be applied directly to the skin, with the exceptions of lavender, which can be applied to burns, and tea tree oils, which can be applied undiluted to insect bites and other wounds. Some aromatherapy oils may already be diluted in a carrier oil and can be directly applied to the skin. Do not dilute further until you have checked the instructions.

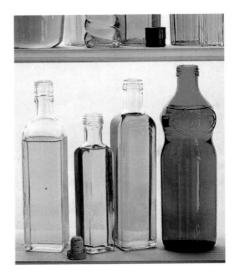

Popular essential oils and their uses

Basil
This oil refreshes and uplifts. It is an anti-spasmodic and nerve tonic and can be used to treat breathing and digestive problems, mental fatigue, stress, and depression.

Black pepper
A stimulating oil, black pepper may be used for clearing catarrh, headaches, food poisoning, and digestive pain. It is also used to treat rheumatism and toothache. Can be an irritant in high concentrations.

Clary sage
A very relaxing, warming oil that can help treat high blood pressure, PMS, menstrual cramps, and depression in women. *Note:* Clary sage should not be used by pregnant women; it may cause miscarriage.

Eucalyptus
A refreshing oil that can clear the head and help treat fluid retention, headaches, and muscular pain. It helps dry up mucus and is used in the treatment of bronchitis and rheumatism. It is also a natural insect repellent and bactericide.

Frankincense
An effective oil that relaxes and rejuvenates at the same time. Known to lift the spirits, it is useful in the treatment of stress and depression and has also been found to be an excellent treatment for boosting the immune system. It may also be used for treating skin problems and cystitis.

Juniper
Depending on your condition and mood, this oil may either relax and refresh you or stimulate you physically. It is a good oil to use if you are under the weather, suffering from cystitis, rheumatoid arthritis, or insomnia. This oil is an anti-inflammatory antiseptic and is useful in treating colitis, enterocolitis, and gastric flu. It is also used in spray form to deter insects.

Lavender
Very useful as an antiseptic. It refreshes and stimulates and is used to treat fluid retention and disorders of the digestive system. It is one of the oils used for labor pains during childbirth. Lavender can also be used in the treatment of burns, infections, and rheumatism *(opposite)*.

Lemon
A stimulating, refreshing oil that is excellent for treating poor circulation, oily skin, and acne. It can be sprayed to act as a disinfectant.

Orange blossom
This very soothing, relaxing oil can help during an anxiety or panic attack. The oil is said to help release worries and so is used to treat stress, depression, and insomnia.

Patchouli
A soothing, relaxing oil that is good for lifting the mood. It is often used to treat or prevent a depressive state of mind and body. It is also useful in treating dry skin. In combination with juniper, cypress, and rosemary, it is used to reduce cellulite because it promotes circulation. It makes a good insect repellent.

Peppermint
A renowned digestive aid that cools and refreshes. It can help treat headaches and motion sickness as well as indigestion and irritable bowel syndrome. It is a good general painkiller and is also used to treat PMS and menstrual cramps.

Rosemary
A must in everyone's medicine chest. You will find this refreshing oil very invigorating. It is helpful for treating bronchitis, physical and mental fatigue, and poor memory. It is also good for sinusitis, bronchitis, the common cold, cystitis, and catarrh.

Tea tree
Another must for the medicine chest—a natural, cleansing antiseptic oil that is excellent for treating insect bites, colds, flu, sinus problems, and sore throats. Its very good antifungal properties help treat thrush and athlete's foot. Use with lavender to enhance the effect and the smell.

Different ways to use aromatherapy

● **inhalation**
Shake 2 to 3 drops on to a tissue or into a small bowl of water in an aromatherapy burner.

● **body massage**
Use 12 to 18 drops per ounce of carrier oil for a body massage.

● **facial massage**
Use only 1 drop of essential oil to 1 teaspoon of carrier oil when using for an aromatherapy facial massage. Avoid the eye area.

● **bathing**
Add 5 to 6 drops of the essence of your choice to make a warm, therapeutic bath.

● **foot bath**
After a hard day's work indulge in a relaxing foot bath by adding 3 to 4 drops of oil into a bowl of water.

● **creams, ointments, lotions, and gels**
Add a few drops to the unperfumed cream, lotion, or gel of your choice. There are also many readymade preparations available.

The healing power of lavender

Lavender is a complete pharmacy in an oil. It is a very special and therapeutic oil that is also useful as an antiseptic.

Use lavender oil in a burner to:
● purify the noxious air in a room.
● purify the atmosphere of a sickroom. Lavender has antibacterial properties. Airborne bacteria are vulnerable to its vapors.
● reduce the tension in a room where you or loved ones are anxious or overexcited.

Use lavender drops to:
● help you sleep at night if insomnia is a problem, or to get you back to sleep if you wake up in the middle of the night. Put a few drops of lavender oil on a tissue and breathe in gently.
● treat burns and sunburn. Lavender can be used either as is for burns or sunburn or you can put 3 to 6 drops in a bath of tepid water.
● treat head lice. Try a mixture of 25 drops each of lavender and rosemary, mixed with 12 drops of eucalyptus or geranium in 3½ ounces of carrier oil. Rub in, leave overnight, and wash out in the morning.
● treat sprains. Add 4 or 5 drops of lavender to a bowl of cold water. Soak a cloth to make a cold compress to help reduce swelling.
● reduce stress. Whether from environmental factors, rush-hour traffic, jet lag, or professional or emotional stress, inhaling lavender oil soothes stress away.
● calm a mother and her unborn child, through massage, inhalation, or in the bath. Lavender is also safe to use on children, as its gentle aroma and unique properties soothe, balance, and relax

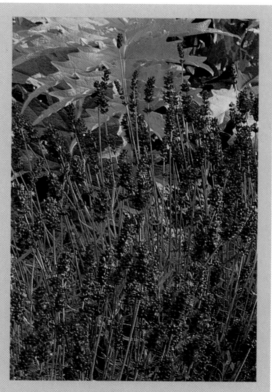

a hyperactive child, or make breathing easier for asthmatic children.
● balance emotions and energy. Whether your feelings are hyper, excitable, flying high, or dulled and depleted, you can use lavender to rebalance your emotions. Drops can be added to a bath, inhaled from a burner, or applied to the skin when blended with carrier oil. You can also put a few drops on a hanky to inhale when you feel stressed.

The benefits of aromatherapy

The combination of essential oils with massage is one of the most powerful, preventive, and therapeutic tools with which to promote and maintain well-being. It has many potential uses:

● It is one of the most immediate, effective treatments for stress. Tensions melt away under the soothing touch of a qualified massage therapist using aromatherapy.

● People with nervous problems respond well to aromatherapy, particularly people suffering from anxiety, depression, and low self-esteem.

● As a beauty treatment, aromatherapy facials can take years off the face by smoothing out wrinkles and softening the tension in face muscles.

Alexander Technique

The Alexander technique is a series of extremely gentle exercises designed to correct posture by realigning the way we use our body. It teaches methods of movement that overcome the potential problems of causing damage to our joints and muscles. The technique was originally developed by an actor, Frederick Matthias Alexander, who realized that the temporary voice problems from which he was suffering onstage were caused by poor posture, particularly tension in his head, neck, and spine. Teachers of the Alexander Technique describe what they do as "an educative process with preventive and therapeutic consequences." Alexander believed that most common health problems are caused or exacerbated by a lifetime's accumulated bad habits in body movement and posture, and so he developed the Alexander Technique to correct negative, compensating patterns of attitude and physical movement.

The technique is usually taught in 10 to 12 sessions, each lasting about one hour. The teachers gently guide you through subtle adjustments in your posture—whether standing, sitting, or lying down—to encourage correct coordination, poise, and alignment. They teach how to change harmful positions, such as slouching in a chair or standing unevenly, into healthy ones and how to use the muscles of the body to maximum effect using minimum effort and strain.

The Alexander technique, however, teaches much more than lessons in deportment. It retrains us to use our body in a healthy and balanced way. By promoting an awareness of the alignment of our skeleton and encouraging an "inner dialogue" with it, it allows optimum relaxation and equilibrium in bones, muscles, and mind. The technique also teaches us how to recondition our mind-body responses and "unlearn" bad habits through self-observation.

Frederick Matthias Alexander

At the turn of the century, Australian actor Frederick Matthias Alexander suffered from a loss of voice onstage, although it returned during periods of rest. He sought help from doctors but conventional medical treatment failed to help him. He was determined to solve the problem and save his career, so he observed himself in a mirror while acting out his part in an attempt to understand what was going wrong. He noticed that as he prepared to deliver his lines and project his voice, he automatically lowered his head, his throat tightened, and his breathing changed. The stress on his neck, throat, and vocal cords was causing him to lose his voice. He began to make a deliberate and conscious effort to change these damaging habits and correct them.

In the course of his self-observation and therapy, he developed the view that mind and body are connected, with one constantly affecting the other. As he further investigated his theory, he evolved a new language of mind-body relationship and a radical way of looking at the effects of negative patterns and habits on both. These became the founding principles of the technique practiced today.

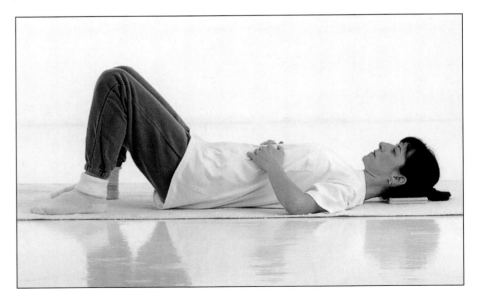

Relaxing the spine
The head is the heaviest part of the body and places considerable strain on the spine. By lying down flat on the floor with your legs bent at the knee and your head resting on a couple of paperback books, you will take the strain off your spine, allowing a natural alignment and relaxation of the skeleton.

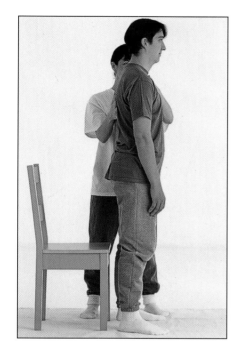 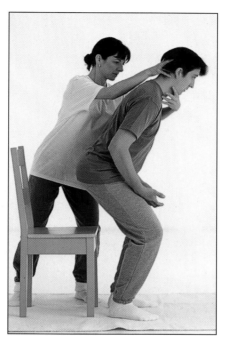 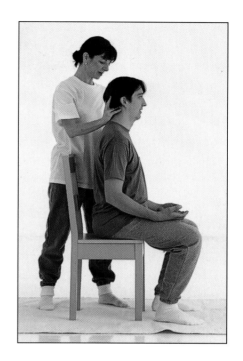

The Alexander Technique is ideal for treating any skeletal and muscular problem and has proved particularly effective in helping persistent back pain. In addition, it promotes a general feeling of well-being that has a positive effect on stress-related conditions such as insomnia and headaches. It is a highly respected technique widely used by many people in the public eye—including singers, actors, and public speakers—because it has such a beneficial effect on posture, voice, breathing, and also on the ability to manage stress.

The Alexander Technique's greatest benefit is less to do with treating already existing problems than with improving health and preventing painful and disabling conditions. Good postural control will help to avoid muscular and skeletal problems resulting from everyday actions such as getting in and out of a car, working at a desk with rounded shoulders—even simply sitting down on a sofa.

Because it is an extremely gentle and subtle manipulative body therapy it is very safe. In addition, it brings about a feeling of overall well-being, relieves stress, and encourages mental and physical balance, poise, and alignment.

To assess your posture, observe yourself in a mirror in the same way that Alexander did. Become aware of how you hold yourself. Do you stand straight and firm but not tense? Are your feet pointed forward and positioned about a shoulder-width apart? Are your shoulders relaxed but not rounded, allowing your neck to be as long, centered, and released as possible? By using the Alexander Technique you can learn how to stretch and relax into your body to achieve greater well-being with the minimum of adjustment and movement.

Alexander movement

This exercise of sitting in a chair will help you become aware of how you use your body. To do it correctly, stand straight, imagining there is a thread running through the center of your body that is being pulled up through the crown of the head. This allows the spine to straighten. Gently bend forward, bending the knees. Now lower yourself into the chair, keeping your back relaxed but straight. You should now be sitting comfortably but with no strain on any of your joints or muscles.

The Alexander Technique can treat:

● arthritis ● backache ● headache ● high blood pressure ● insomnia ● postural problems ● repetitive stress injury (RSI) ● respiratory conditions ● rounded shoulders ● stress ● tension ● tight neck ● tight throat ● voice problems.

Acupuncture and Reflexology

Acupuncture—literally "needle puncture"—is a healing technique that involves inserting fine needles into the skin. It is an integral part of traditional Chinese medicine, a complex, 5,000-year-old system of healthcare that also includes diet, exercise, and the application of heat and herbal treatments.

The technique involves inserting needles along the meridian (energy) lines of the body in order to boost their pathways to promote good health. The use of acupuncture for pain relief is renowned. In the West it has proved extremely helpful during labor, where its pain-relieving properties have the advantage of not affecting the baby. In China it is widely used instead of conventional anesthetics for both minor and major surgery. As it tends to induce feelings of relaxation and general well-being, it is an excellent technique for treating any stress-related disorders, depression, anxiety, and tension. It has also proved successful in treating addiction, such as assisting smokers in quitting cigarettes.

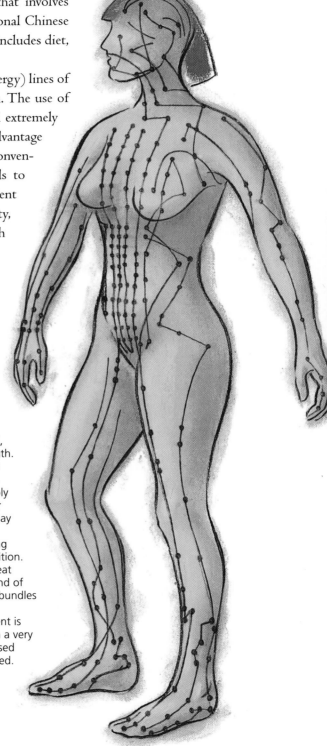

The Chinese believe that the body is governed by various meridian (energy) pathways that control different parts of the body.

Diagnosis and treatment

An acupuncturist diagnoses an affected organ and assesses your internal energy in a number of ways, including visual inspection, paying careful attention to what you say and taking notes on your health history. The two main techniques, however, are pulse and tongue diagnosis.

The practitioner feels the pulse near the wrist, checking its speed, rhythm, strength, and regularity. There are many different variations and an experienced practitioner can distinguish between them to diagnose an imbalance. The tongue is thought to mirror the body's condition and examining it is an important diagnostic technique in all forms of traditional Chinese medicine. It is worth noting that taking Western drugs can adversely affect the accuracy of the acupuncture diagnosis.

Once the practitioner locates the meridian that needs rebalancing, he or she selects one or several acupuncture points. A needle is inserted into the chosen point to a depth of only a fraction of an inch. (A needle may be inserted as deep as three or four inches in some parts of the body.) Most people do not feel its insertion, although sometimes there is a slight tingling sensation. At the beginning of a course of healing, the needles are left in for only a few minutes, but later they may be left for up to 30 minutes. Their removal is also painless and bleeding is very rare. Acupuncture needles are made from stainless steel, are very fine, and vary in length. Properly trained practitioners *always* use sterilized needles.

The practitioner may simply leave the needles in place for a specific length of time or may twirl them to stimulate the acupuncture point, depending on your symptoms and condition. For additional stimulation, heat may be applied to the free end of the needle by burning small bundles of herbs.

A more recent development is electroacupuncture, in which a very small electrical current is passed through the needle that is used.

The laws of Yin and Yang

The Chinese believe that the entire universe, including human beings, is subject to the laws of Yin and Yang. These refer to ch'i–or natural energy–an invisible, powerful force in everything, from the air we breathe to the water we drink, as well as the life force in our bodies.

Yin energy is female, receptive, soft, dark, and negative. Yang energy is male, creative, hard, bright, and positive. A balance of these opposing energies produces harmony, wholeness, and good health. Maintaining this equilibrium is essential to well-being.

The vital energy, ch'i, flows through the body along 14 main paths, known as meridians. If the flow of ch'i is blocked or disturbed in some way, this will affect an organ on that specific meridian, even though it may be located some distance from the blockage. There are many different acupuncture points along each of these meridians where the flow of ch'i can be stimulated and the balance corrected by the insertion of the needles.

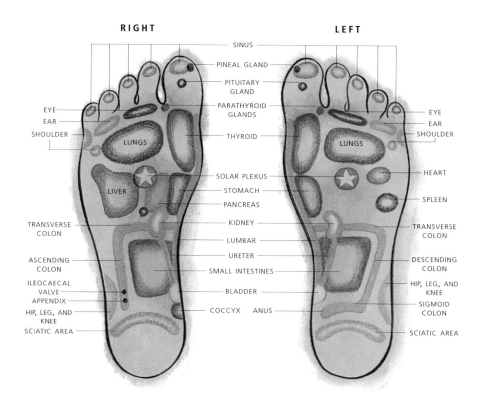

RIGHT — LEFT

SINUS, PINEAL GLAND, PITUITARY GLAND, PARATHYROID GLANDS, THYROID, SOLAR PLEXUS, STOMACH, PANCREAS, KIDNEY, LUMBAR, URETER, SMALL INTESTINES, BLADDER, COCCYX, ANUS

EYE, EAR, SHOULDER, LUNGS, LIVER, TRANSVERSE COLON, ASCENDING COLON, ILEOCAECAL VALVE, APPENDIX, HIP, LEG, AND KNEE, SCIATIC AREA

EYE, EAR, SHOULDER, LUNGS, HEART, SPLEEN, TRANSVERSE COLON, DESCENDING COLON, HIP, LEG, AND KNEE, SIGMOID COLON, SCIATIC AREA

Reflexology

Also known as zone therapy, reflexology is a massage treatment that concentrates on specific areas on the soles of the feet, stimulating, pressing, and kneading them to bring health and well-being to other parts of the body.

Reflexology stimulates the immune system and recharges your personal powers for self-healing. The therapy is based on the belief that energy flows through channels in the body and an imbalance or blockage of this energy results in disorder and disease. Reflexologists divide the body into 10 zones, each of which corresponds to an area on the soles of the feet; the toes, for example, correspond to the head. Specific organs are thought to be linked to these zones via the nervous system.

By stimulating the nerve endings in the appropriate place on the soles of the feet–the reflex point–a reflex response is caused in the relevant organ. For example, a reflexologist would massage the tops of the big toes to relieve and treat migraine headaches. The left foot mirrors the left side of the body and the right foot the right side.

A reflexologist will spend some time examining the soles of your feet and, perhaps, giving them a gentle overall massage to diagnose any problems. Any areas that are painful or tender are likely indicators of specific organs that will benefit from treatment. He or she will also probably consider your health history and look out for general signs of stress, pain, or muscular tension.

Having identified the appropriate treatment points, the reflexologist will apply firm pressure, mainly with the thumb, to relieve tension and to rebalance the body. This is rarely uncomfortable, but you may experience feelings of sensitivity, tenderness, or even ticklishness. Reflexology using essential oils is becoming increasingly common.

As it has no known side effects, reflexology is a popular therapy for treating many disorders. For the same reason, it may also be used as a complementary therapy to any conventional treatment. Its effect is soothing and relaxing, so it is ideal for eliminating stress. It may also be useful in protecting health and preventing illness.

Accurate diagnosis by a properly trained reflexologist can indicate areas of potential weakness that, if left untreated, may potentially lead to more serious problems later on.

Cleansing and Detoxing

Cleansing the inner and outer body is an effective way to improve health. It helps rid us of the dirt and pollutants that find their way into the lungs and bloodstream and cling to the skin and hair. It can jump-start a metabolism that has become sluggish through poor diet and speed up the removal of toxins and biological debris that build up in the lymphatic system. On top of all this, it suffuses us with a wonderful feeling of well-being and renewal.

Cleansing rituals such as fasting and the washing of feet have played an important part in cultures throughout the world for thousands of years. The Romans took cleansing very seriously. Their methods were nothing if not thorough: Visitors to their communal baths oiled their bodies and entered a series of chambers with rising degrees of dry or steamy heat. Dirt, oil, and sweat were then removed with a special scraping tool known as a strigil. The heated communal baths sometimes contained health-giving minerals and there was often a cold plunge pool.

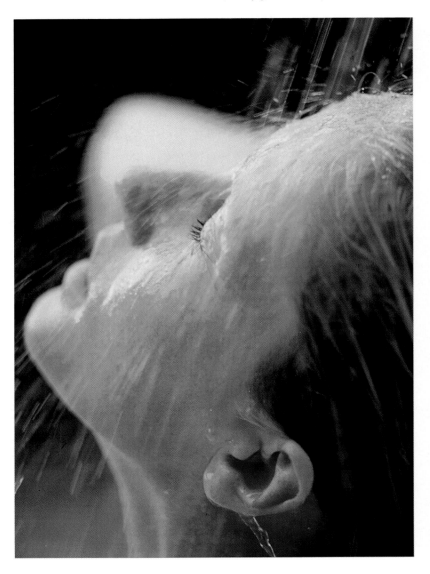

The refreshing, cleansing power of water not only keeps us clean but helps pep up the circulation, bringing blood to the surface of the skin and a clean, healthy glow to the body.

Even today our own varied cleansing techniques using bath oils, body scrubs, saunas, and steam baths remain remarkably similar. Many methods of deep cleansing, such as saunas and Turkish baths, rely on alternating hot treatments with cold. This makes them very effective at toning the circulation. In addition, there is a theory that intense heat stimulates the immune system in much the same way as a fever. The heat opens the pores, softens any plugs of sebum blocking them, and encourages profuse sweating. Tiny blood vessels beneath the skin's surface dilate and the circulation slows, allowing more nutrients from the blood to diffuse into the cells. The cold water treatment that follows causes the pores and arteries to contract to conserve heat. This boosts circulation and the extra warmed blood surges deep into the body. So despite the cold, you end up with an intense warm glow, very similar to that experienced after vigorous exercise.

Bathing

Baths can be relaxing or invigorating. You can choose the mood you want to create by swishing a few drops of an appropriate aromatherapy oil into your bath water. Lavender and neroli oil promote relaxation, while lemon grass, lemon, and petitgrain are refreshing. Alternately, add about a quart of an infusion of dried herbs to your bath. Try exquisitely scented dried lemon balm, elder flowers, crushed cardamom seeds, lime blossom, or chamomile.

Magnesium-rich Epsom salts or a cup of cider vinegar added to the bath water relieves aching muscles. For sensitive skin, soothing oatmeal—on its own or mixed with dried marigold petals and wrapped in cheesecloth or muslin—proves an excellent soap substitute and gentle exfoliator. Sea salt is a more effective exfoliator that efficiently polishes away rough skin, while olive oil massaged all over before a bath loosens dead cells and leaves dry skin feeling luxuriously moisturized.

Clay-rich mudpacks and mud baths exfoliate by absorbing dead skin cells and excess sebum, making them perfect for oily skins. Seaweed and algae wraps are claimed to be diuretic, which is why they are often recommended for those who suffer from water retention. Sea minerals, extracts, mud, and aromatherapy oils may also be incorporated in hydrotherapy treatments that claim to be able to help reduce cellulite.

Detox diet

An extremely effective way to cleanse your inner body is through a three-day detoxification diet. It not only energizes, but you may well find that minor health problems like acne, dull skin, constipation, and headaches—often symptoms of a toxic overload—vanish afterward. Eating light meals of easy to digest raw, fresh fruits and vegetables, rich in fiber, vitamins, minerals, and other nutrients, will help cleanse the colon and flush out the kidneys.

Start the day with a glass of warm water with slices of unwaxed lemon or a cup of herbal tea, sweetened, if you prefer, with honey. Drink copiously throughout the day, but never an hour before or after a meal so your digestive juices remain undiluted when they have to break down food.

Drink uncarbonated mineral water, freshly squeezed fruit juices, and two or three cups of powerfully diuretic celery seed tea. (Use I teaspoon of culinary seeds per cup, as sowing seeds are often treated with fungicides.) If you experience a caffeine withdrawal headache, drink a cup of strong chamomile tea to relieve the discomfort.

Enjoy a large plate of fresh fruit for breakfast and always eat slowly, chewing each mouthful thoroughly. For lunch, have a large salad bowl of any vegetable you fancy, sliced, grated, chopped, or eaten whole. Finally, eat another large plate of fruit for your evening meal.

Spend your time resting, reading, and listening to soothing music or relaxation tapes. If you like, practice some gentle stretching exercises, yoga, or meditation.

Repeat on day two and three, although substitute your final meal on day three with a light water- or vegetable stock-based soup made from a purée of any green vegetables you like and a teaspoon of vitamin- and mineral-rich Japanese miso paste. Over the next few days just eat some light meals that incorporate plenty of fruits and vegetables.

Clean out your system by eating a diet of fresh fruits and vegetables. They have a high water content, which helps them pass quickly through the kidneys and colon, flushing out waste as they go.

Colonic irrigation

The process of flushing out the digestive system by colonic irrigation has grown in popularity, although medical opinion is still debating the possible benefits.

During colonic irrigation fluids are passed into the colon via a tube inserted through the anus. The fluid, which is essentially warmed water, is then passed back out again, carrying any matter in the rectum and colon out with it.

Those who support this practice believe that this method cleans the intestines, eliminating stored fecal matter, gas, mucus, and toxic substances. Practitioners claim it helps with constipation and detoxifies the body. Others believe that it is harmless and ineffective.

A process similar to colonic irrigation is performed by advanced practitioners of yoga, who look on it as an important purification process.

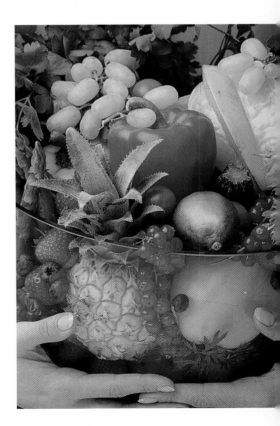

Seasonal Boosters

With electric light, central heating, modern greenhouse horticulture, and fresh vegetables now jetted into supermarkets from all over the globe, the changing seasons fail to make as much impact on our lives as they must have done to our forebears. Nevertheless, the seasons still exert a powerful influence on us. Scientists have discovered that in spring, as the temperature rises and the hours of daylight extend, testosterone levels rise in men and women. This promotes that "get up and go" feeling as well as boosting our sex drive. Summer is an easy, relaxed time, when we enjoy the good feeling the sun brings. The sun also increases our vitamin D levels. As the nights draw in during autumn, the natural tendency is to withdraw and become less active. When winter finally arrives, lethargy can have set in and our bodies feel sluggish. But we can feel good all year round by acknowledging the changes in the seasons and making a commitment to maintain a healthy lifestyle.

Seasonal changes

To stay in top form all year round, we need to adapt our lifestyle to meet the challenges of each season.

Winter

With modern insulated homes we no longer need to burn up extra calories just to keep our bodies warm, and since we are also far less active than our great-grandparents, we need fewer calories than they did. The watch point for winter is diet: We need to lower our fat and sugar intake and eat more fruits and vegetables. Supplements of vitamin C are wise because fruits and vegetables stored over the winter lose some of their vitamin C content. Eating plenty of garlic, which has antibacterial properties, should reduce the risk of respiratory infections.

If you do feel a cold coming on, you may be able to ward it off with a 20-minute mustard footbath. Stir a tablespoon of ordinary mustard powder into a deep basin of the hottest water your feet and lower legs can comfortably bear. A few drops of ginger and juniper oil added to a carrier oil or body lotion rubbed into the skin will also warm and revive you when you feel chilled.

The other essential is to remain active. Brisk winter walks are excellent for toning up sluggish systems. Getting out in the crisp air and daylight improves your mood, too. With the pressures imposed by the holiday season to cope with, it is also essential to incorporate some form of relaxation into your life. Yoga or tai chi are particularly recommended because they keep joints and muscles flexible in cold weather as well as calming the mind.

Spring
This is the perfect time to clean your inner body with a detoxification diet (*Cleansing and Detoxing, page 84*) to get rid of the wastes that have built up over winter. Make the most of fresh green leaves that are rich in protective antioxidants such as beta carotene, vitamin C, and iron—like spinach, spring greens, and watercress. If you have put on weight over the winter through inactivity, consider taking up a

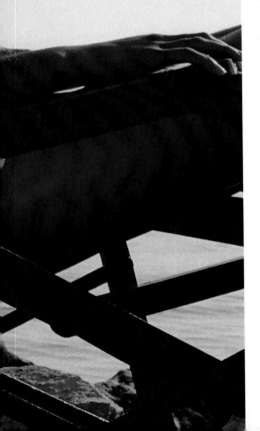

new sport. Now is the perfect time to get active as you have the whole summer season to continue to improve your fitness. Treat dry, chapped winter skin by exfoliating and then massaging in coconut or almond oil. Supplements of starflower or evening primrose oil help dry skin, too.

Summer
This is the time to make the most of the great outdoors, providing you maintain a healthy respect for the dangers of the sun. UVB rays are linked with skin cancer and UVA with premature aging, so wear a UVA/UVB sunscreen whenever you are out for any length of time. All sunscreens carry a Sun Protection Factor (SPF) rating. This rating is a guide to how much UVB protection a sunblock offers. For example, if you can remain in the sun for 15 minutes before burning, the SPF rating on a sunscreen is simply the figure you multiply by 15 minutes, to find out how much longer you can stay safely in the sun after applying that particular sunscreen.

There are serious doubts about the safety of tanning beds, so a better way to give yourself some healthy-looking color is by using one of the much improved "indoor tanning" products now available. Risking skin cancer by using a tanning bed is foolish in the extreme.

Summer is the perfect time to take up swimming, aqua-aerobics, or any other water sport. They are all excellent, all-around ways of improving stamina, strength, and suppleness.

Autumn
Resist the temptation to slow down—try to remain active. If you find you are losing interest in outdoor aerobic activities as the temperature falls, switch to an indoor aerobic exercise like skipping, using an exercise bicycle, or aerobic exercise classes.

Fruits, and vegetables are still plentiful, so eat a wide variety and try to continue eating salads at least two or three times a week. Switch to a slightly richer moisturizer, body lotion, and hair conditioner to combat the aftereffects of the sun and to prepare for the ravages of winter weather.

Seasonal Affective Disorder
There are people who become depressed every year as the days start to shorten and who don't cheer up until the spring. No one knows how many people suffer from this seasonal depression, which is widely known as seasonal affective disorder (SAD). It was once thought that the problems experienced by SAD sufferers were psychological in origin, but research has shown that it may actually be a strong sensitivity to lack of light that makes sufferers depressed.

SAD is now a recognized condition that affects four times as many women as men and is most common in the 20 to 40 age group. If winter brings on a touch of the blues, then a regular dose of full-spectrum light could put you back in the pink.

Light is the visible part of a spectrum of energy of differing wavelengths. Daylight is made up of the full spectrum of primary colors, but artificial light has shorter wavelengths in a narrow band of the light spectrum.

Despite justifiable concerns about long-term exposure to the sun, a little sunshine is definitely beneficial. Sunshine provides the full-spectrum light that is essential to our well-being and health. In the summertime, when full-spectrum light is easily available on sunny days, the symptoms of SAD disappear—and do not surface again until the onset of winter's short, gray days. Although some people may need antidepressants to combat SAD, you may want to try these aids: Take noontime walks; set your bedside lamp to turn on an hour before you normally get up; get plenty of exercise; ignore any cravings for high-carbohydrate junk foods; and maintain a well-balanced diet.

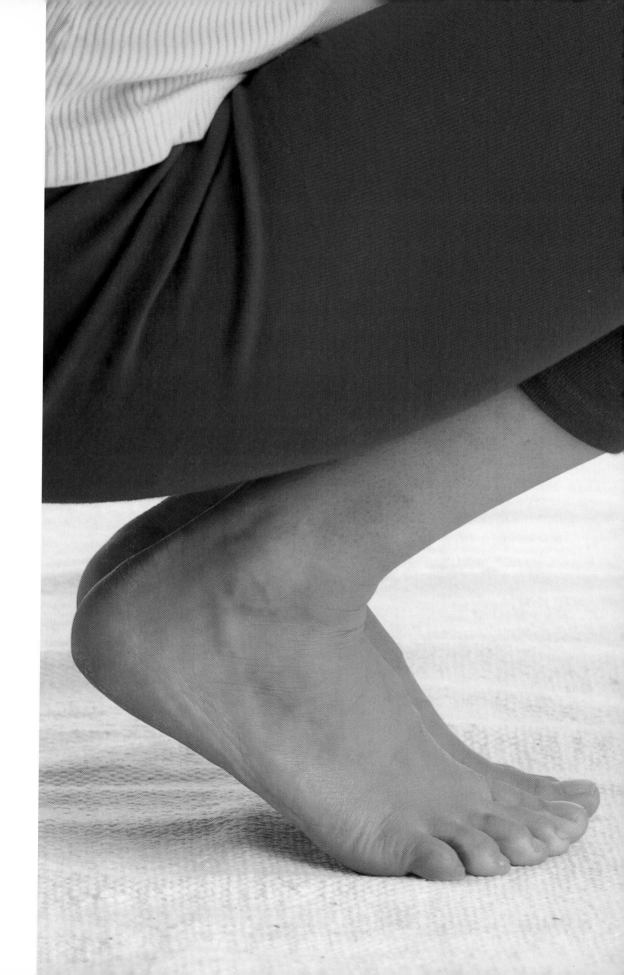

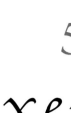

5
Exercise for Health

The real key to achieving optimum health and well-being in the stress-filled world that we live in is to exercise regularly. There is more to good preventive healthcare than eating a balanced diet, taking vitamin or mineral supplements, or treating ourselves regularly to an enjoyable natural therapy such as a massage. Regular exercise is the primary solution to many of the health problems facing us today.

At the beginning of human evolution our bodies were designed for activity. From hunting and gathering to visiting or exploring, we walked or ran everywhere. However, in this century modern technology and the car took over.

Increasingly, health experts around the world attribute the huge rise in the incidence of diseases, such as heart disease, to our sedentary lifestyle and lack of regular exercise, as well as to a diet too high in fat.

By regularly exercising with sports or dance three to four times a week we can tone and condition our muscles and bones, and achieve a healthier body and mind.

The Importance of Exercise

To keep your body looking and feeling good, two of the most important things you can do are to eat a good, well-balanced diet and exercise regularly. Most people know that they should have regular exercise, but all too often they do very little about it. It is easy to come home tired after work and just slump in front of the television rather than play a sport or go to an exercise class. But if you make the effort to exercise, even for a short time, you will soon feel the benefits. After exercising you will find that your tiredness or tension headache has miraculously disappeared and that your spirits have lifted. You will feel more positive about your life and experience a kind of exhilarating "high" as your body releases endorphins—the body's natural pleasure hormones.

The reason we have to think consciously about incorporating exercise into our day-to-day lives is that we have become so inactive. In our grandparents' day there were fewer cars, and people would often walk or cycle miles to get where they needed to go. Nowadays, most people drive everywhere. If you are short of time, it is so easy to jump in the car and drive to the mall, even if it is only a short distance away. Our jobs have also become much more sedentary. With the integration of computers into office life, many of us can now spend several hours a day sitting in front of a computer terminal, hardly taking a break. So it is not surprising that we often get home feeling tired and lethargic.

If you are moderately fit already, the current recommendation to keep healthy is to do at least 20 minutes of vigorous exercise, such as running, cycling, tennis, squash, or aerobics, three times a week. But recent research has suggested that if you are unfit, you can still benefit, at any age, by doing 30 minutes of moderate exercise (so that you feel slightly out of breath) five times a week. Swimming or walking are ideal low-risk exercises to start with.

Don't exhaust yourself by rushing into a heavy exercise program. In the first month just do 30 minutes for one day a week and then build up gradually. You need not change your lifestyle greatly to do some moderate exercise. Try walking instead of driving. Walk up the stairs at work, rather than using the elevator. Or get off the subway or bus one stop earlier and then walk briskly the rest of the way to the office.

If you can't easily play tennis, or get to a dance or yoga class, you can still keep fit with shorter and more frequent periods of exercise. Decide what is best for you. If your regular two to four sessions of exercise a week make you feel great, stick with it—but work in different ways of toning your body every so often.

Exercise does not always have to be strenuous; walking (right) is one of the most beneficial forms because it conditions the whole body.

Driving is essential to many of us nowadays, but it is also very sedentary. To get more exercise leave the car at home for short journeys and walk instead.

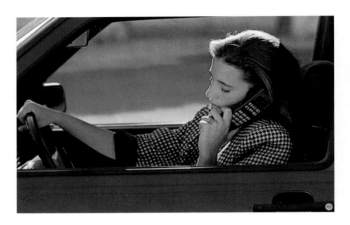

Benefits of different exercises

Once you start regular exercise you will soon notice the improvement in your body shape and how it:

- Reduces the risk of heart disease.
- Improves your circulation.
- Improves your breathing and your entire respiratory system.
- Helps alleviate symptoms of osteoarthritis.
- Increases bone density, lowering the risk of osteoporosis.
- Strengthens your back and reduces lower-back pain.
- Strengthens muscles, tendons, ligaments, cartilage, and stabilizes joints.
- Increases flexibility.
- Slows down the aging process.
- Increases energy.
- Helps reduce body fat levels.
- Helps maintain ideal body weight.
- Improves digestion.
- Helps correct bowel problems, particularly constipation.
- Improves self-esteem and body image.
- Reduces depression, anxiety, and stress.

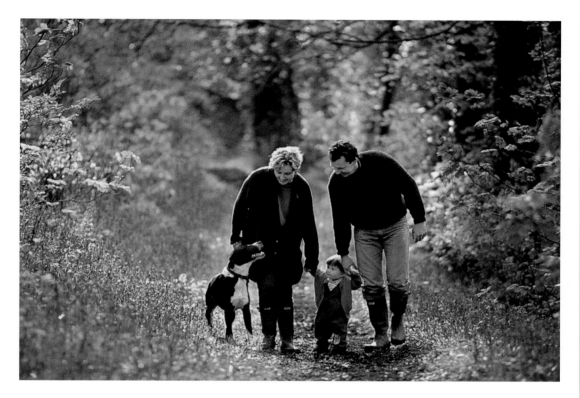

No matter what type of exercise program you choose, there are some important rules to consider before you start:

● Warm up before exercising by stretching your muscles.

● Gently stretch your muscles again as you cool down.

● Allow yourself to go slowly and gently, no matter what exercise you do.

● Aim for gradual progress in your physical achievements.

● Breathe evenly and deeply when exercising, exhaling breath for that extra effort or stretch.

● Work at your own level and pace. Do not try to keep up with those who are fitter.

● Listen to your body and stop exercising if you feel faint or experience pain.

● Be aware of your posture; keep your shoulders down and your tummy pulled in.

Improving your body

As stress has become such a regular factor of our daily lives many people have started to look for activities that calm their minds as well as work their bodies. The oriental arts of yoga and tai chi are less aggressive forms of exercise that involve both the mind and body. The mind is first slowed down by the use of deep-breathing techniques, tension is released, and the body is then exercised by slow stretching and controlled body movements. This type of exercise is suitable for older people.

Once you start to exercise regularly you will soon feel the improvements to your body. By becoming fit your body will gain suppleness, strength, and stamina.

Suppleness will give you more flexibility and mobility in your neck, trunk, and limbs. With exercise the joints become tightened and toned up and the supporting ligaments are in turn shortened and also strengthened.

Strength is the muscle power that you need for pushing, lifting, and moving things around. This is developed by exercising body muscles against some form of resistance such as cycling up a hill or using weightlifting equipment. Exercised muscles, including the heart, become bulkier and stronger.

Stamina is the staying power your body gains. When you increase stamina it means that you can continue a muscular activity, such as running and swimming, for longer without getting breathless. You also improve your body's cardiovascular performance by getting your body to work aerobically—your lungs and heart work hard, your breathing is increased, and your blood circulation is stimulated.

Increasing the amount of exercise that you do can help you maintain your best weight. It also reduces the risk of developing high blood pressure or heart disease and helps prevent the onset of osteoporosis, a disease—mainly affecting postmenopausal women—in which the bones start to lose calcium and become very brittle.

You will find that regular exercise helps your mind. It increases your energy level and vitality while also letting you wind down and relax, so that you forget the stresses and strains of your busy working day. The deep-breathing techniques you adopt during exercise will also tone up your nervous system. Finally, by looking good physically, you will become more confident in yourself and you will start to project a much more positive mental outlook in all aspects of your daily life.

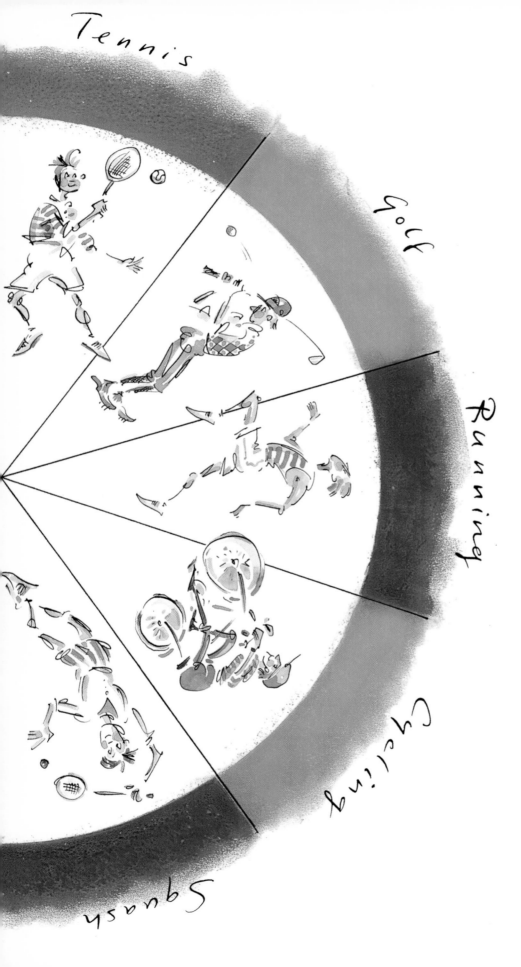

Tennis

Golf

Running

Cycling

Squash

Choosing an exercise

There is a rich and varied selection of exercise systems from which to choose the best exercise/fitness program for your needs and circumstances.

The way we exercise is as individual as the way we eat, sleep, or relax. When choosing an exercise, what matters most is that you are engaged in an activity that feels good to you and is appropriate to your age.

If you have a history of regular participation in any sport such as running, cycling, swimming, tennis, golf, or squash, or other movement systems such as dance or gymnastics, you are likely to be in good shape. If you haven't exercised for a long time, are generally unfit, or are recovering from illness, there is still a form of exercise for you—tai chi and yoga are very safe, low-injury-risk exercise systems.

To choose the exercise that is right for you, follow the exercise wheel. Identify the sport you are particularly interested in and check whether you are up to that level of fitness by matching up the shading with the fitness shading guide. This will tell you if you are at the correct level—not very fit, moderately fit, or extremely fit—or how to assess which level of fitness you would like to achieve.

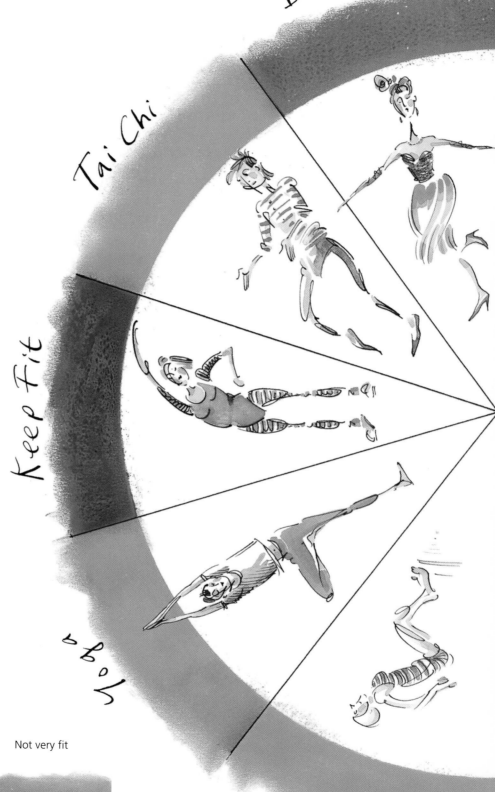

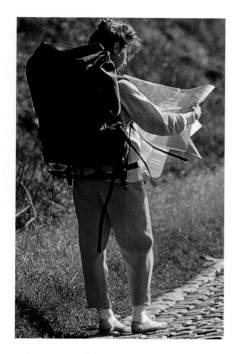

Hiking is an outdoor pursuit that you can consider undertaking if you are moderately fit (you already do some form of exercise). Since the emphasis is so much on your legs in this form of exercise, it is worth considering doing some leg strengthening exercises in a gym before you start. You will need to build up body strength and stamina through another sport or movement because hiking can involve trekking up and down difficult terrain for long periods of time.

Ballroom Dancing

Tai Chi

Keep Fit

Yoga

Swimming

Shading:

Extremely fit   Moderately fit   Not very fit

Sports and Dance

Once you have decided to take up an exercise routine, or increase what you do already, you need to investigate what type of sport or dance will suit you. You also need to think about your current fitness level. If you occasionally attend an aerobics class and walk a lot you should be reasonably fit and could consider engaging in a vigorous sport such as squash or circuit training in the gym. However, if you rarely exercise and find you easily get breathless walking up stairs, you are better off starting with a less energetic regimen, such as walking or yoga.

If you decide on an aerobics, fitness, or dance class, seek out your nearest class. You can then either buy yourself workout clothes or just wear a T-shirt and shorts or sweats. Good training shoes are important. Consult your local sports shop about the different styles available, especially for step classes. If you prefer a racket sport, choose a nearby club: You will not keep the sport up if you have to travel miles to play. For squash and badminton, you will need a racket and appropriate athletic shoes.

A skiing holiday is fun, but you should build up stamina before you go, and renting equipment is expensive. Walking is the cheapest way to increase fitness. You can wear any comfortable clothes, but make sure you have a good pair of walking shoes. Before taking up a vigorous sport, have a physical examination.

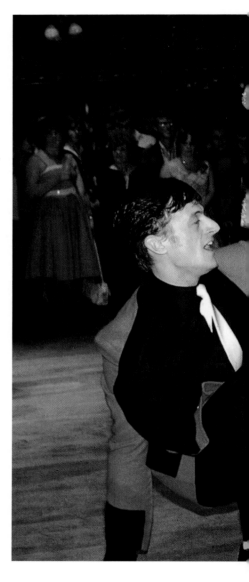

Benefits of different sports

Tennis: Tones muscles, increases suppleness. Generally anaerobic exercise. Good for hand/eye coordination.
Suitable for: All age groups, some basic fitness necessary. Good social sport.

Badminton: Increases flexibility and stamina; tones muscles. Normally anaerobic exercise, but can be aerobic when played hard. Can help prevent osteoporosis.
Suitable for: All age groups, some basic fitness necessary. Good mixed sport.

Squash: Vigorous anaerobic sport. Tones most muscles and increases flexibility. Improves racket/eye coordination.
Suitable for: All age groups with good fitness levels; not suitable for unfit or overweight people, or people with heart conditions or joint problems unless under a doctor's supervision.

Golf: Some muscle toning in arms and shoulders. Can improve balance and co-ordination. Brisk walking over a course can help improve cardiovascular fitness.

Suitable for: All age groups, but particularly the over-50s; golf is not too strenuous. Good social sport.

Aerobics: Good all-around cardiovascular workout. Tones all major muscles in the body; increases suppleness and stamina.
Suitable for: Most age groups, but high-impact level suitable for young people and low-impact for the over-40 age group.

Cycling: Strengthens and tones legs and buttocks, and to a lesser extent the arms and shoulders. Increases cardiovascular fitness; improves stamina.
Suitable for: All ages. The overweight benefit from cycling slowly. Not advisable for people with respiratory problems.

Swimming: Ideal all-around body exercise, supported by water. Strengthens cardiovascular and respiratory systems, builds stamina, tones muscles.
Suitable for: All age groups, even the elderly. Good strengthening exercise for people with bad backs or injured muscles.

Riding: Works all body muscles, particularly calves and thighs. Helps balance.
Suitable for: All age groups, but not advisable for people who have suffered head injuries or have joint problems.

Skiing: Strengthens and tones leg muscles and buttocks. Improves balance and agility.
Suitable for: People of most age groups with good fitness levels. Good social sport.

Dance: Builds endurance and agility. Increases stamina and suppleness.

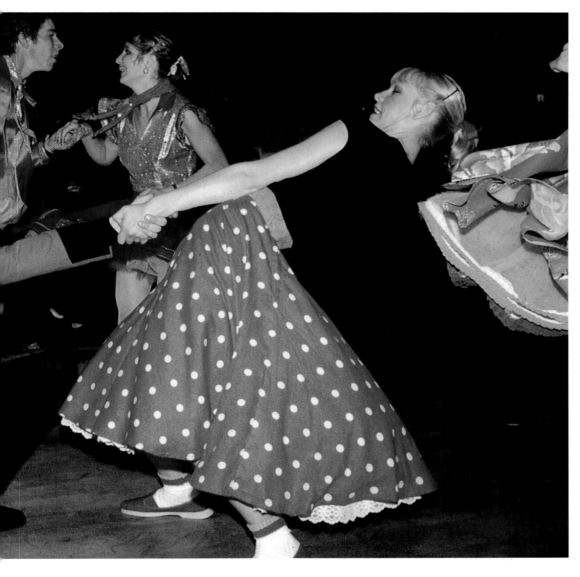

If you go to an energetic dance class, such as one that involves rock music, you will increase your cardiovascular endurance and also tone and strengthen your arm and leg muscles. You will also find that your body becomes much more supple.

Suitable for: All age groups, although disco dancing appeals to the young, while ballroom dancing is for mixed age groups.

Tai chi: Slow, deliberate exercises and regulated breathing calm the mind, release tension, and improve concentration. It also increases body flexibility and suppleness.
Suitable for: All age groups, even the unfit.

Yoga: Relaxes body and mind. A series of slow, stretching movements with deep, controlled breathing help to improve

suppleness, stamina, and muscle strength, while clearing the mind. Builds confidence.
Suitable for: All ages—even those who are unwell can benefit, provided a trained yoga teacher supervises their exercises.

Circuit training (in the gym)**:** Routines to increase stamina and strength and to tone muscles; ideal complement to skiing and tennis. A circuit should also include aerobic exercise such as cycling or swimming.
Suitable for: Young people with good fitness levels.

Running: Good for cardiovascular fitness, muscle toning, and weight loss. Can also have psychological benefits.
Suitable for: All age groups with good fitness levels.

Fitness: Aerobic sessions improve cardiovascular endurance, while body conditioning exercises tone and strengthen muscles and improve overall suppleness.
Suitable for: Young people with good fitness levels, although less energetic classes are available for the over-50s.

Martial Arts

Most of the martial arts that are popular today have their origins in Japan or China. They were developed as an ancient means of self-defense and unarmed combat, using kicks and punching movements, and in their original forms were brutal and often lethal. They also contained mental and spiritual training, however, that gave the contestants amazing control over their aggression and fighting movements. Over the years they have been refined into controlled combative techniques that are extremely useful in self-defense, but that draw on powerful concentration and meditative techniques to complete the moves.

The main combative martial art forms practiced today are judo, karate, and aikido, which involve kicking, throws, pinning movements, blocking skills, grappling, and joint-locking techniques. Tai chi is one of the oldest Chinese martial arts: It has studied movements practiced more for fitness than combat.

The combative martial art forms are quite vigorous. They can be undertaken by people of most ages, but participants must already have some degree of fitness. Classes are held in sports centers and martial arts clubs. Students wear loose-fitting suits tied with belts. Normally there is a grading system, indicated by the color of the belt worn. As the student improves, a higher grade and a different colored belt are earned. A one- to two-hour session once a week is the minimum training that is recommended. If you have knee, elbow, or lower-back problems consult your doctor before taking up a martial art.

Regular participation in martial arts gives the body a good cardiovascular workout and helps develop muscle tone, strength, and flexibility. The whole-body exercise can help to maintain bone density and control weight and body fat. Balance and concentration are also improved by controlling the set movements. Coordination improves and the body moves more quickly, increasing agility with the fast actions. The body and mind become focused together when using the techniques.

With the noncombative martial arts the main benefits are in general health and well-being. The more meditative approach to the movements helps relax both the body and mind, slowing down breathing, improving mental concentration, and increasing body suppleness.

The different art forms

Karate (Art of the Empty Hand)
This martial art has many forms. It originated in Okinawa during the 16th century, when Japan was occupied by the Chinese and forbade the inhabitants to carry any weapons. Modern-day karate was first introduced by Funakoshi Gichin in 1922 when he staged exhibitions and tournaments for the Japanese public. Karate actions consist mainly of striking, kicking, and blocking skills. Karate quickens responses as well as giving the body a good, all-around workout.

Judo (Way of Gentleness)
This ancient combative martial art was once known as jujitsu. Since its adoption by the Japanese military and police it has been called judo. It was founded by Jigoro Kano, a student of jujitsu who started a judo center in Tokyo in 1882. Judo involves throwing, grappling, strangling, choking, and joint-locking techniques. Its aim is to defeat the opponent, either by throwing her onto her back for 30 seconds or by securing submission using an armlock or another technique. With regular practice judo improves all-around fitness, helps to give the body a good cardiovascular workout, and increases overall stamina levels. Some of the falls in judo can be heavy, so particular attention needs to be paid to falling correctly to minimize the impact on the body.

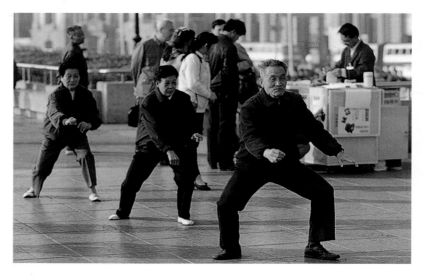

Tai chi, the ancient Chinese martial art, is now very popular in the West. Its gentle meditative technique helps to relieve stress and relax both the body and mind.

Aikido (Way of Spiritual Harmony with Energy)

Founded by the religious master Morihei Ueshiba in the early 1930s, this martial art has its origins in jujitsu but was also inspired by the 13th-century style of daito-ryu. Aikido involves body throws, pins, joint leverage techniques, and weapons training. There are two main styles of aikido–ueshiba and tomiki–with the latter style involving a competitive element. The benefits of aikido are similar to those of judo and generally improve all-around fitness.

Wu shu kwan (Chinese kickboxing)

Most of the techniques of this ancient combative Chinese art form are verging on gymnastic, which has implications for the performer's fitness and health. Similar to kung-fu, kickboxing involves a wide range of fast kicking movements against an opponent. It gives modern practitioners good self-defense skills, helps improve muscle strength and flexibility, improves speed and agility, and develops concentration and confidence. It can also help with weight control.

Tai chi (Supreme Ultimate Fist)

Also known as tai chi chuan, this ancient martial art was first practiced in China some 5,000 years ago. The techniques and flowing exercises, coordinated with controlled breathing, are performed in an unhurried, meditative manner and are practiced to improve fitness rather than for combat. Tai chi relaxes both the body and the mind, releasing tension and making individuals focus on their bodies and breathing. With practice, one movement flows easily into another, unconsciously helping the body to achieve more flexibility and suppleness. A great deal of concentration is required in the art to develop the necessary mental control and to calm the mind.

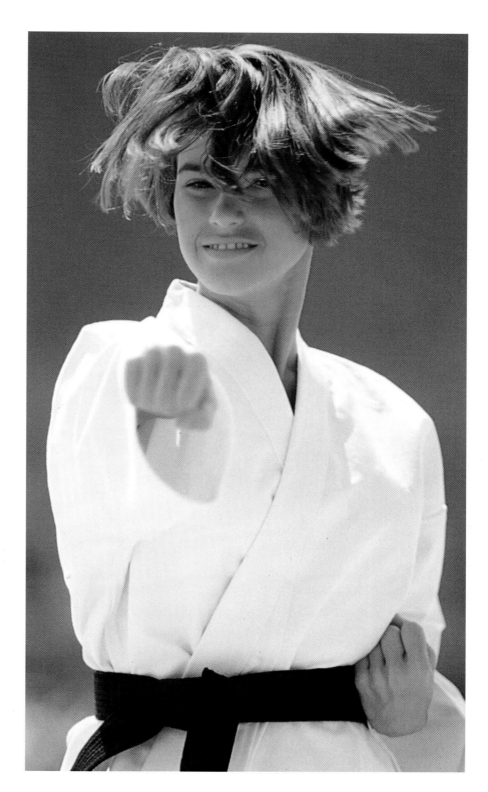

Women can become more assertive and gain more self-confidence from learning a martial art, such as judo or karate. With practice, they can also acquire some useful self-defense movements.

Yoga

For thousands of years the peoples of India have practiced the holistic system of exercise known as yoga. In more recent years, people all over the Western world have learned the simple, powerful techniques of yoga and have experienced the benefits of this ancient body-mind-spirit culture.

The word "yoga" means "union" and the exercises can teach you how to restore balance and suppleness to your mind and body through a series of breathing exercises and physical postures. By practicing yoga you not only stretch and tone your body but also learn how to relax the mind, dramatically improving your powers of concentration. The aim of yoga is to bring the body and the mind into a state of perfect equilibrium by practicing a series of physical, mental, and breathing exercises that lead to a state of optimum well-being on every level.

Broadly, yoga can be divided into two areas: Hatha yoga, which develops the physical body through a series of asanas, or postures as they are often called, and other yogas like Karma, Bhakti, Jnana, and Raja, which focus more on the meditation process in relation to your work, devotional life, mental processes, and spiritual life. All the different yogas are integrated with pranayama–the science of breathing according to yogic teachings.

In their book *Yoga and Health,* yoga experts Selvarajan Yesudian and Elisabeth Haitch state: "this system is unique in the entire world, since it consciously perfects the body, compensates for any physical defects, and fills it with glowing life force. Hatha yoga leads us back to nature, teaches us about our own body and the forces acting within it, and leads us to the close harmony of body and soul."

Learning yoga increases your body awareness, suppleness, and strength, as well as your sense of well-being. The first thing you will need to master before you learn the postures is how to stand properly. You need to become aware of how to distribute your weight evenly on both sides of your body while standing, using proper breathing techniques, and encouraging the right body alignment and balance.

When practicing yoga or any other exercise system, it is important to find a qualified instructor who will teach you how to do the movements correctly. Equally important is having the right mental attitude: Leave any competitiveness behind; never force yourself past a point of pain; listen to your body and your breath, take it slowly and gently; and try to keep your concentration focused on what you are doing.

Lesson 1: Tadasana–good posture
Stand up straight with your feet together. Do not lock your knees. Place equal weight on both legs. Keep your pelvis tucked in and let your shoulders relax downward. Close your eyes and focus your attention on your spine and the symmetrical alignment of your entire body. Stand in this relaxed manner, holding a good posture for several minutes.

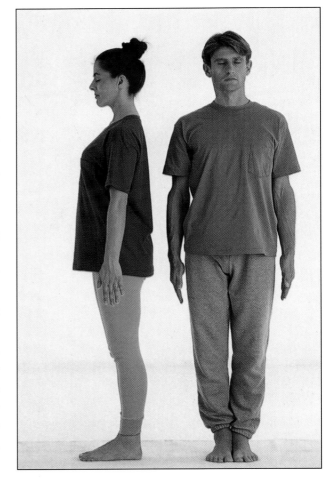

A true awareness and mastery of good posture—Tadasana—provides a firm foundation to build upon. The standing postures strengthen and tone the leg muscles, feet, and ankles, as well as the spine and abdomen. By learning to stand firmly on the soles of the feet, you can relieve stiffness in the leg and hip muscles and strengthen your stomach and back muscles, enabling the hip joints and spine to be more mobile. This is the first step toward reaching full flexibility.

Some of the standing postures help you widen and lift the chest and upper back areas and correct round shoulders. This in turn enables you to breathe more deeply and to balance yourself with greater ease. Standing positions can improve posture and blood circulation.

When you ignore the force of gravity on the body and your left and right sides are unbalanced, your nervous system suffers. Correcting posture by practicing the standing positions alters your psychological as well as physical state, and you begin to feel lighter in your body and more agile in your mind. By gaining a sense of balance and poise you will feel true equilibrium and general well-being.

Relaxation poses that involve lying on the floor can calm your mind and really release tension from your body.

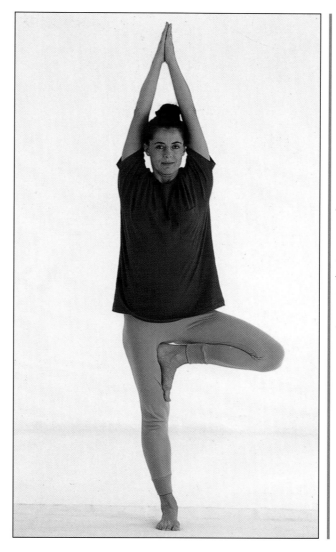

Lesson 2: Tree pose

This simple standing posture teaches you how to balance properly. Start by standing upright and practice a few rounds of deep yoga breathing. Focus on a spot on the wall in front of you around eye level. Inhale deeply and place your left foot on your inner right thigh, keeping your right leg straight. Exhale as you bring your arms in front of you, put your palms together, and then raise your arms above your head, keeping your elbows straight. Breathe evenly and concentrate on balancing for 20 to 30 seconds. Then exhale deeply, bring your arms and leg down, and repeat with the other leg.

Lesson 3: Savasana— relaxing pose

Lie on your back with your feet slightly apart. Put your arms at your sides with your palms facing upward. Extend your trunk, arms, and legs, and then relax them. Close your eyes and breathe in and out deeply.

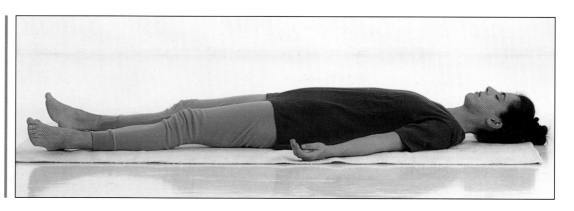

Salute to the Sun

In yoga, after learning how to properly stand and relax, one of the first sets of asanas you learn is called the Salute to the Sun exercise (Soorya Namaskar). This exercise is a combination of yoga asanas and breathing actions that help build a strong and flexible spine and limbs. It can help to reduce your weight, increase lung capacity, and provide the perfect warmup for practicing other yoga postures.

The Salute to the Sun exercise is made up of 12 spinal positions that stretch the vertebral column and its various ligaments. The 12 positions make up one full round of Soorya Namaskar. Do the exercise once or twice to start with, and slowly build up until you can do the exercise 12 times without straining yourself too much. Some people may never feel comfortable doing it more than three to six times. Always listen to your body when doing any form of exercise. There is a very fine line between pushing yourself and overdoing it.

Be careful not to strain or push yourself too far or too fast when doing any of the positions. Also, it is always a good idea to take instruction from a professional yoga teacher in the early stages of your practice—just to be sure you learn the correct and safe way to do the basic postures.

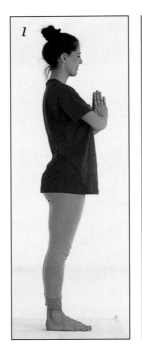

Step 1
Stand in an upright position with your feet together. Put your hands together in front of you in a prayer position. Keep your palms touching; make sure your fingers point upward.

Step 2
Inhale slowly and deeply, while raising your arms above your head. Then gradually bend backward, pushing with your arms.

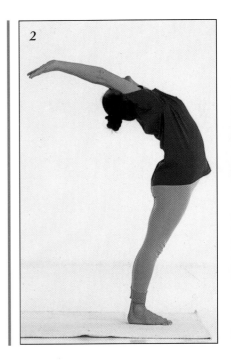

Step 5
Inhale again and hold your breath. Move your left leg back from your body to line up with your extended right leg. With your feet together, lift your body off the floor, balancing on your straight arms and toes. Keep your body in a straight line.

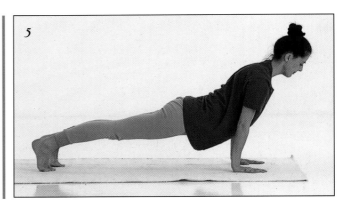

Step 6
Exhale slowly while you gradually lower your body down to the floor, bending your arms. Make sure your knees, chest, and chin are in contact with the floor.

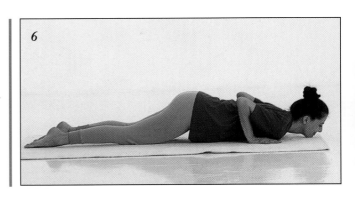

Step 3

Exhale slowly and deeply as you bend forward to hold on to your ankles or to touch the floor. Remember to tuck in your head as you bend. To begin with, you may find it easier to bend your knees in this step, but as you develop more flexibility try to straighten them.

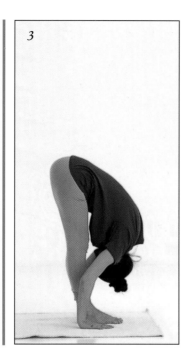

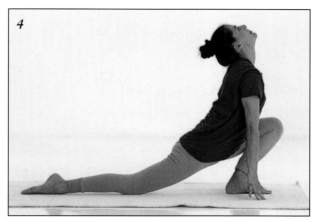

Step 4

Inhale again and move to a crouching position. Keep your left knee bent and slide your right leg behind you in a big step. Keep your hands and left foot firmly on the ground. Once your right leg is in position, gently bend your head backward as far as it will go to stretch out your spine. Exhale.

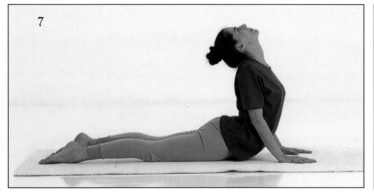

Step 7

Inhale slowly and deeply as you lift your trunk upward and bend backward as far as possible, leaving your lower abdomen, pelvis, legs, and hands firmly on the floor. This movement is similar to the Cobra position in yoga.

Step 8

Exhale and lift up your buttocks and back. Tuck your head in and keep your feet, heels, and hands flat on the floor.

Step 9

Inhale, crouch down, and balance on your right knee, extending your left leg behind you. Lift your head gently backward, slightly bending your spine back as in Step 4.

Step 10

Exhale and bring your left leg forward again. Crouch down, lift your buttocks, and clasp your ankles as in Step 3.

Step 11

Stand up straight and inhale, raising your arms over your head and bending gently backward as in Step 2.

Step 12

Exhale, lower your arms. Repeat 1 to 11 times.

The Well-Being Fitness Plan

This program is suitable for people who are completely new to exercise. The plan should, if followed regularly, help to give you more stamina and muscle tone. It will also make you more flexible, and can help you to lose weight.

It consists of four sections. First is Warming up, to ensure that your muscles are loosened up and ready to work harder. This is followed by the Cardiovascular workout. Cardiovascular, or, aerobic, activity will get your heart pumping faster and increase the flow of blood to the muscles. This section can also be structured to ensure that you burn fat throughout. Conditioning is a series of exercises designed to tone up the major muscle groups, while also involving the biceps, triceps, calves, and other smaller muscles in the body. Finally, the Cooling down section will, if followed properly, allow your body to adjust from higher levels of activity and reduce the likelihood of strain or soreness occurring, as well as increase your overall body flexibility.

There are varying levels of intensity described as the program progresses, and you should follow all the instructions closely. Keep your breathing deep and regular throughout, and note the safety hints on page 104.

Each exercise is explained in words and pictures. Always start gently at the easiest level, and increase the duration as you become comfortable with the exercise and the techniques.

Warming up

Using the heart rate chart on page 104, take your resting heart rate before you start any exercise session; you can compare that rate with the levels that you reach during the session. Try to devote five minutes to the initial warmup, easing into each stretch without straining or bouncing, and holding it for 30 to 40 seconds.

Stretch gently at first, concentrating on the major muscle groups—chest, thighs, hamstrings, and back. You should also try to run through these stretches after you do the vigorous Cardiovascular workout. By then you will be a lot more flexible, as warm muscles stretch much more effectively than cold ones do, and you may find it easier and more comfortable to hold each stretch for that little bit longer.

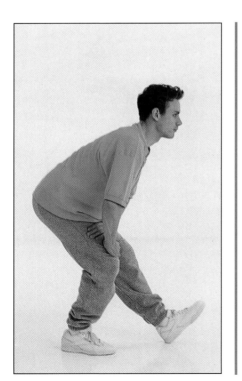

The hamstring stretch
This exercise is designed to stretch the hamstring muscles at the back of the thigh (left). Stand on your right leg with your right knee slightly bent. The left leg should be straight and stretched out in front of you with your left foot flexed. Put your arms on your right leg and gently bend from the hips over your left leg until you feel the stretch at the back of the left thigh. Change legs and repeat.

The thigh—quadriceps—stretch
Stand on your right leg, ideally supporting yourself against a wall or chair with your right hand. Keeping your right knee relaxed, grasp your left foot with your left hand near the ankle, or closer to the toes to stretch the shin muscles too (right). Gently pull your left foot up toward your buttocks to feel the stretch in your thigh. Change legs and repeat.

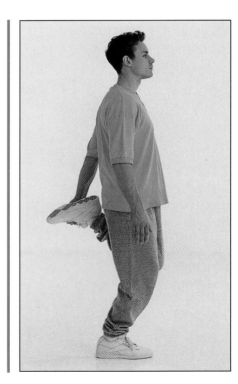

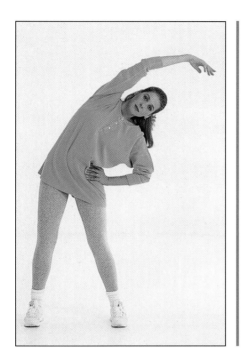

Side stretch

Stand with your legs just over a hip-width apart with your knees relaxed. For an easy stretch, put both hands on your hips and bend over to the left very gently until you feel a stretch along your right side. To increase the intensity, put your left hand on your left hip to support your body weight and lift your right arm above your head and bend over to the left again (left). Change sides and repeat.

Chest stretch

Stand looking straight ahead with your right hand on a wall beside you with your fingers turned out behind you (right). Turn your head and body to the left and feel the stretch across the front of your chest and in your right arm. Change sides and repeat.

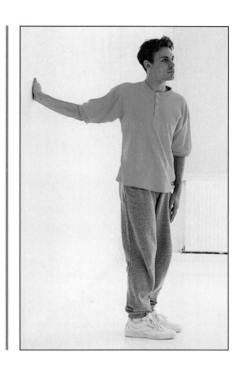

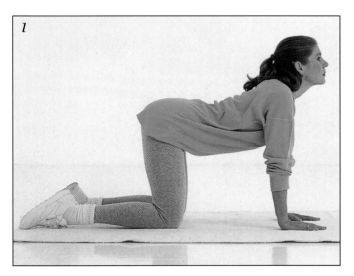

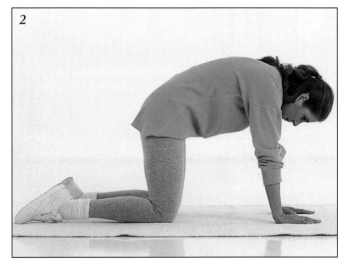

Back (Cat) stretch

Go down onto your hands and knees (1). Keep your arms and legs slightly apart and make sure that your knees are aligned beneath your hips and that your hands are beneath your shoulders. Keep your hands flat on the ground with your fingers facing forward and spread apart. Lift your head up and hollow out your back gently. Hold this position for 30 seconds.

Now gently reverse the exercise, moving your head downward to look at the floor, rounding your back as you do this and stretching it upward (2). Hold this position for 30 seconds, then repeat each move to really feel the stretch in your spine. This exercise helps to loosen you up and will release tension in your back, particularly if you are deskbound.

Timing

You should aim to go through this fitness plan, which takes about an hour, at least three times each week. You can increase the duration of each session by adding a longer cardiovascular workout, and by spending more time stretching at the end–stretching will greatly benefit you later in life, by keeping your joints supple and mobile.

The number of times an exercise is performed is called a repetition. A set is the number of repetitions that you do. Most of the conditioning exercises start with four sets of 10, and increase over time to four sets of 15 before you should increase the intensity. Aim to add one repetition on each set at every session, if you are consistently exercising three times a week or more. Space your sessions out over the week. Four sets is a lot for absolute beginners, who may find that just one set is enough. For those who cannot commit themselves to such a schedule, try to add one repetition every four sessions if this feels comfortable. Keep a record of when you exercise and the number of sets/repetitions that you do, or the length of time it took to do the cardiovascular workout, to assess your progress.

Safety hints

This program is intended for healthy people. If you are not fit, please consult your doctor before starting to exercise. This is important if you have a medical condition, past or present, or are taking medication that could affect your training ability. If you ever feel dizzy or nauseated during a workout, stop immediately and consult your doctor.

• Always wear comfortable clothing–workout clothes or shorts and T-shirts, with good training shoes that fit properly.
• Regularly drink water throughout the workout to rehydrate yourself.
• Do not eat 2 to 3 hours before an exercise session.
• Breathe deeply and regularly during a workout, and always make sure you breathe out as you exert effort.
• Always stretch at the beginning and end of the session as this will help to keep your joints supple and mobile.

Cardiovascular workout

This section will give your body a good cardiovascular workout, help you to burn fat, and will also exercise your heart and lungs. Your initial workout should take 5 minutes and you should then progress at 30-second or one-minute intervals until you have reached a regular, manageable session of 20 to 30 minutes of intense aerobic activity.

It is useful to measure your pulse rate while you are exercising by pressing your index and second fingers against the carotid artery in the side of your neck or on your wrist. Do this at regular intervals throughout your workout, and try to ensure that you keep to the target ranges for your age group *(chart, below)* for the duration of this section.

Choose a cardiovascular activity that you enjoy, and feel free to mix and match different activities across the duration of the program. For example, you could do 10 minutes bouncing, 15 minutes fast walking, and 5 minutes of skipping if that is what you want to do, as long as you watch your pulse and keep to the training range that you have set.

If you regularly use a gym you can divide your workout between the cardiovascular machines that are available there. For example, you might want to start with 10 minutes on a bike, then do 15 minutes on a step machine, and end up with the last 5 minutes on a running or a rowing machine.

Heart rate chart

Regularly checking your pulse rate when doing cardiovascular exercise lets you know that your heart and lungs are working efficiently. Check your pulse (at the neck or inner wrist) and count the beats for 10 seconds (first beat 0) and then multiply by 6 to give your pulse rate per minute. This will give you a figure that you should compare with the target heart rate based on your age.

You should be aiming to achieve between 55 and 75 percent of your maximum heart rate output. If you are using a machine, such as a bike, with resistance levels and you are peaking above or below your recommended heart rate, adjust the level up or down to suit.

Target Heart Rate Zone Chart

Age	Ideal beats per minute
15–19	111–154
20–29	105–150
30–35	101–143
36–45	96–138
46–55	90–130
56–65	85–123
66 and over	80–109

Walking or running

These activities are the simplest form of aerobic exercise, and they require little or no practice! Make sure that you always walk safely: Don't walk in places that are deserted or dangerous if you are alone. It is also unwise to walk on your own wearing headphones. Try to exercise within your target heart rate (chart, left) at all times. It is easy to amble along for 20 minutes, but this won't do you much good other than getting some fresh air. Your foot should strike the ground heel first, with the pressure moving to the ball of the foot. Start with a brisk five-minute walk, and increase the pace and distance gradually. If you want to run, try running for 30 seconds, then walking for 30 seconds over a 5-minute period, increasing the running periods when you feel comfortable.

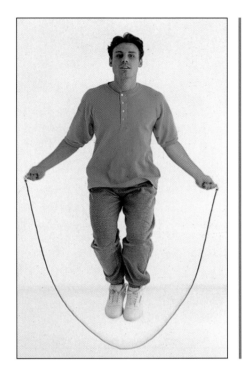

Skipping

Skipping rope is an intense cardiovascular exercise that can be surprisingly tiring, and it is probably better for those with some cardiovascular strength (left). It requires little equipment or space. Use a good rope (leather ropes are the fastest) and try it before you buy it to ensure that it works well and is right for you. Find a smooth surface on which to skip and, since skipping is a high-impact exercise, preferably one with a little give, such as a sprung wooden floor, to avoid damage to joints. Start skipping for a couple of minutes to get used to the motion. Start with slow skipping, where both feet leave the ground together and you do a small skip in between jumps, and then progress to faster, one-jump skipping without the small skip as you become more confident and more proficient in your skipping action.

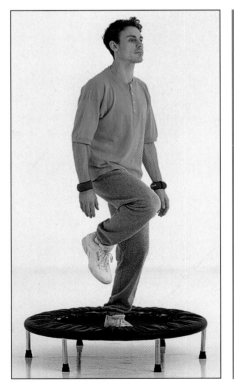

Bouncing

This is another exercise that requires little space and minimal equipment. Trampolines can be bought from most good sports stores and are a good low-impact form of exercise. Start with simple bounces, with both feet together, keeping your arms slightly out to the side to help you balance. As you become more comfortable, increase the tempo of your bouncing, and add in some arm movements to increase the effect. Try bicep curls, keeping your elbows at your sides, and curling your hands up to your shoulders, or chest presses with your hands at shoulder height, pushing out from your shoulders in front of you or above your head. You can bounce from one foot to the other as you gain confidence, and add light hand weights to make it harder. Start with 5 minutes at a low intensity and build up to 20 minutes of bouncing. Stop slowly and dismount carefully as the ground has a habit of coming up to meet you!

Conditioning

Once you have adapted to your cardiovascular routine and started to burn fat, you can move on to this conditioning section, which helps you to tone your muscles and condition your body. Each exercise has specific instructions that you should follow closely, particularly when you first start the program. Position yourself carefully and breathe deeply during each exercise to get the best results. There are ways in which you can increase the difficulty of each exercise, and again these are clearly detailed. Always pace yourself properly, and do not attempt to do the most difficult version of an exercise first, as you may well strain or stretch a muscle, or injure yourself more severely.

Press-ups

This is a good all-around exercise for your shoulders, chest, and upper back. Start on your hands and knees, in the same way as the cat stretch (page 103), but with your hands placed just outside shoulder width (1). Bend your elbows so that your shoulders, chest, and face come toward the floor. Try to create a 90° angle at the elbow (2), then push yourself up again. Do four sets of 10 of these, and progress to 15 repetitions per set before you move on to the next version.

In the next version you lift more of your body weight. Start on your hands and knees but with your knees moved back so there is a straight line from your shoulders through to your hips and your knees. Again, start with four sets of 10, and gradually increase to 15 per set. If it is more comfortable, cross your ankles and bring them toward your buttocks, so that you are resting on the more fleshy part of your knees. Finally, if you feel strong enough, you can do a full press-up: Start on your hands and feet with your legs straight out behind you so there is a straight line from your shoulders to your feet. Keep your back straight as you go up and down, but stop when you are tired.

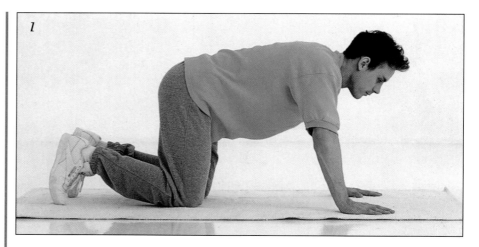

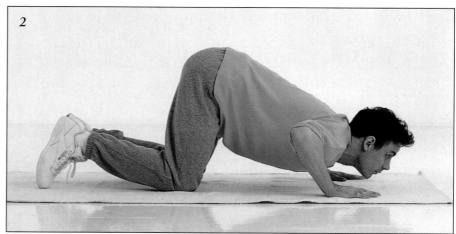

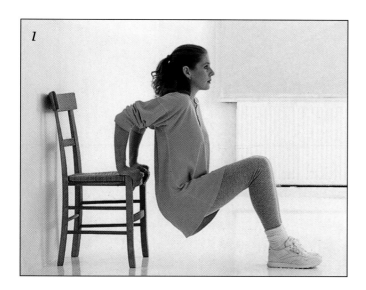

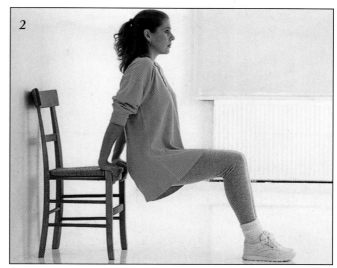

Triceps dips

This exercise strengthens and tones your shoulder, back, and upper arm muscles. Sit on the edge of a chair secured against a wall. Put your hands by your hips with your fingers curled over the chair's edge. Place your feet a short distance from the chair and then, breathing in, lower your body, with your elbows behind you, toward the floor (1). Hold briefly, then raise yourself up again as you exhale (2). Do four sets of 10 repetitions, then increase to 15. To make it harder, move your feet farther out. Then do four sets of 15 repetitions with only your heels on the floor and your legs stretched out.

Abdominal crunches

Lie on a mat on the floor with your knees bent and your hands supporting the back of your head (1). Start first with the simple version of this exercise. Keep your elbows back, and push your lower back into the floor, while pulling in your stomach muscles and lifting your shoulders off the floor (2). Do four sets of 10 repetitions and work up to 15 as you improve. Your neck muscles should become accustomed to the strain as you pull up and down, but at first you may feel some discomfort unless you support your head properly. Do not pull your head forward because you might strain it. Imagine that you have an orange tucked under your chin; keep that posture throughout the exercise. To increase the intensity of the exercise, raise your feet off the floor and bring your knees toward your chest as you raise your shoulders from the floor.

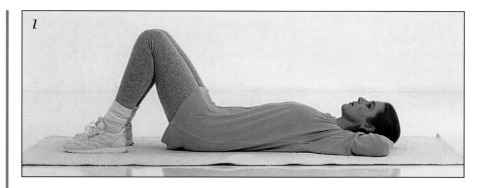

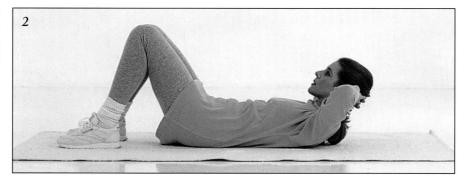

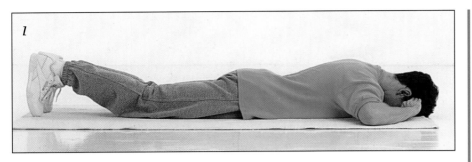

1

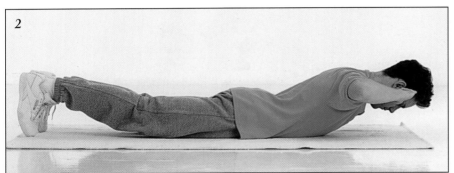

2

Back lifts

Lie flat on your stomach on a mat on the floor with your legs straight but your toes pointing downward toward the floor. Start with the simpler version (not illustrated) and link your hands together behind you at the small of your back. Raise your torso up as far as you can, feeling the muscles in your lower back and buttocks contracting as you do so. Lower your body again. Do four sets of 10 repetitions, increasing gradually to 15 repetitions. To intensify this exercise, lie in the same position but hold your hands at the side of your head (1). Pull your torso up off the floor but keep your feet on the floor so you do not overextend yourself (2). Lower your body again, keeping the movement slow and controlled.

Lunges

This exercise is excellent for the quadriceps and gluteal (buttock) muscles. Keep a good posture throughout.

   Start with a box or step about five inches high in front of you. Step onto the box with your left leg (1). As you start to lunge, make sure the knee of the left stepping foot stays above the ankle, while the right knee almost touches the ground (2). Do 10 lunges with the left leg, then change to the right and do 10 lunges on that side, followed by a further 10 lunges per leg, alternating the left and right legs (20 steps altogether). Increase these to 15 on each foot, and 15 alternating lunges, over a period of time as you feel comfortable. Try to ensure that your back stays straight and strong throughout each set of exercises, and does not bend forward.

   As you start to get stronger, you can increase the intensity of the exercise by carrying some light hand weights, as shown,

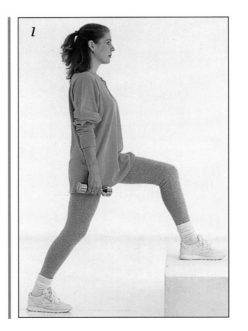

1

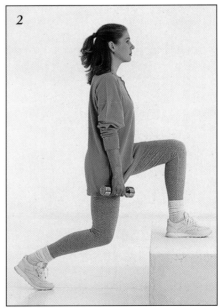

2

or by removing the box. Keep lunging forward, using a smooth, steady rhythm. Make sure you are using strength rather than momentum to keep the movements

going. Breathe in deeply as you go down into each lunge and remember to breathe out as you push yourself back up into a standing position again.

Squats

Stand with your feet slightly apart, and your toes pointing forward (1). Start to squat, bending your knees and pushing your arms forward, ensuring that the weight of your body is supported on your heels, not your toes (2). Slowly push up again from the squat and repeat 10 times, for four sets. Increase this slowly to 15 repetitions. Do not squat any lower than knee height because you might strain your knee joints. You can intensify the exercise by adding light hand weights, as shown, holding them in both hands and thrusting them out in front of you as you squat.

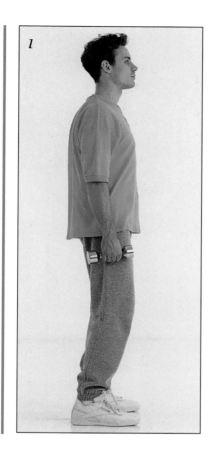

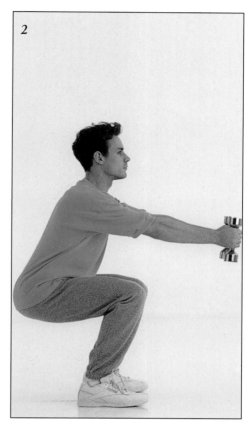

Cooling down

Cooling down is just as important as warming up. You should never stop abruptly after exercise without giving your body the opportunity to adjust to a slower pace. Go through the same stretching exercises as detailed in the Warming up section on pages 102–103 to cool down. The stretches should be held again for about 30 to 40 seconds each time, but you can hold them for longer if it helps to relieve the tiredness in your muscles.

Keep a note of how long it takes your heart to get back to its normal resting rate *(chart, page 104)*. As you start to get fitter, this time should become shorter and shorter, and it is a useful way of measuring an increase in your level of fitness.

Conclusion

You may find that after a few weeks of fitness training you notice a difference in the way your clothes fit you, but that you actually weigh more than before, especially if you are not dieting. This is because muscle weighs more than fat; do not worry about it.

The percentage of your body weight that is fat helps to indicate health: the lower the fat, the better. Muscle burns energy (calories) faster than fat, so the more muscle you have developed, the faster you will burn calories.

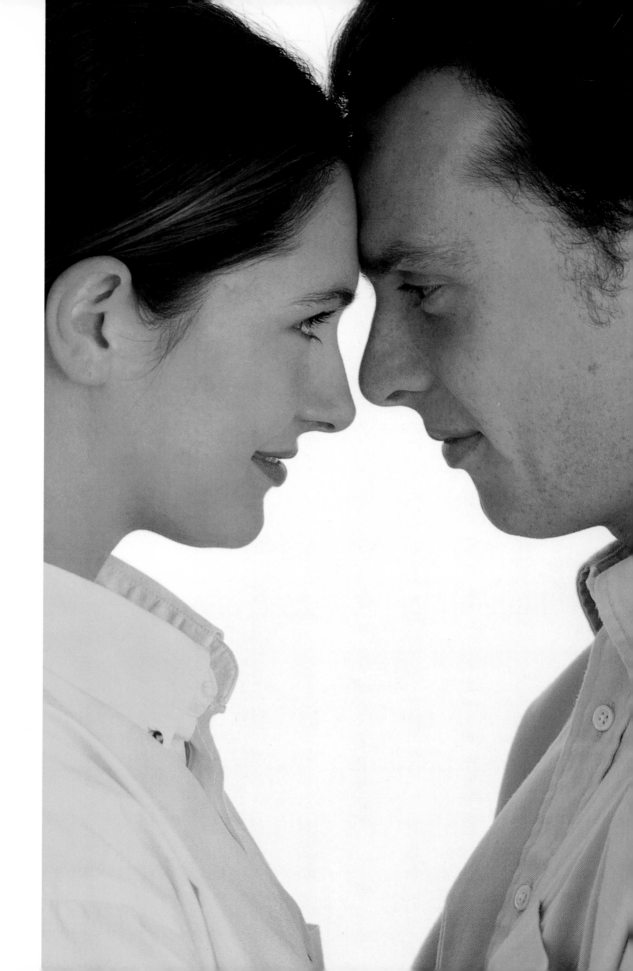

6
The Well Mind

A healthy, balanced mind is something we should all aim to achieve and not take for granted. It is very difficult in our busy lives to keep our minds in shape. We think we have everything on an even keel and then another crisis occurs that throws us into despair. But there are ways to control the stress that continually affects us, and if a critical event occurs that is too much for us to cope with, counselors are available to help guide us through it.

Personal happiness and general self-confidence are also very important to our well-being. These can be enhanced by having the right outlook and attitude.

It is now widely recognized by experts everywhere that the mind and body relationship is intricately interdependent and that one cannot be healthy without the other. It is possible to learn how to keep the mind healthy and acquire different skills and techniques to reach a more balanced and stable mental state, without which a happy and fulfilling life is not possible.

Stress

Stress is the spice of life. Without some new challenges, some uncertainty, or some pressure, our lives both at work and at home would seem rather dull. But stress is often seen as something that needs to be beaten or avoided, and it has been singled out as a cause of heart attacks, substance abuse, and sleepless nights.

Of course too much stress can damage us. Feeling overworked and out of control does make people ill, and people vary enormously in the levels of stress they can tolerate. The constant demands and pressures that top politicians or show-business stars thrive on would quickly drive more ordinary people to drink heavily or to have a nervous breakdown. The secret of having a healthy, balanced life is to keep stress at a level that you can cope with.

Whether the type of stress experienced is positive or negative, it has the same effect on the body. It triggers the arousal system, which starts up as soon as something unfamiliar or threatening happens. The muscles tighten, the blood supply to the surface of the skin is reduced, action hormones are pumped around the body, and the heart starts to beat faster. The body is experiencing a typical "fight-or-flight" response.

How you interpret this explosion of physical energy is what decides whether you call it stress or excitement. If you are a trader on Wall Street, or work as a PR executive, you will probably take the fight reaction, regularly using and enjoying the energy for application, assertiveness, and high endeavor. But if you are working in an office and you're reacting in this way because of the actions of a bullying boss or an impossible schedule, that's when you will probably experience the flight reaction, feeling you can't cope and wanting to distance yourself from the pressures. In this situation you can also freeze and suddenly be paralyzed by indecision, anxiety about your position, and feelings of self-doubt.

Being energized positively and then being able to relax afterward is fine. Problems start to occur when you can't solve the problems or switch them off. When you experience the flight or freeze response for several days or weeks at a time, your immune system may become depressed and you may get sick. Modern office life, where people are constantly working under pressure, seems to be designed to create ongoing low-level stress. Surveys show that many workdays are lost to illnesses caused by job-related stress.

But it is not just the office that can cause stress. Major life events, such as getting divorced, the death of a loved one, moving to a new house, or starting a new job, can all be very stressful. The key to keeping your life balanced is to notice when problems are affecting you, to take steps to control them, and to calm yourself. With long-term problems you need to try the relaxation techniques detailed in Chapter 7.

Handling long-term stress

The key to dealing with the stress in your life is to avoid what is often known as Type A behavior–being aggressive, impatient, and competitive. Try to practice some of the Type B characteristics by acting in a more relaxed manner and not being so anxious about deadlines. Use some of the tips on the opposite page to relieve stress, then try some of the techniques below:

• Make a list of the activities that cause Type A behavior in you. If waiting in line makes you impatient, then next time you are in a long line at the supermarket think of something pleasant.
• Make sure you have enjoyable pastimes: Play a musical instrument or paint.
• Create time for yourself. Take a long, relaxing aromatherapy bath or read a good book.
• Get regular exercise. Two or three 20-minute periods a week of strenuous exercise will help relax tense muscles.
• Eat a healthy diet and take vitamins B and C when you feel you are under stress.

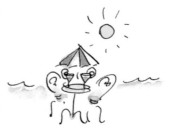

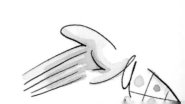

Stress-related illnesses

Many studies have shown that when people are suffering from severe stress their immune system works less effectively. Students studying hard for exams or recently bereaved people are all more likely to catch infections. Even minor conditions, such as headaches, backaches, abdominal pains, and anxiety, can be associated with stress. And conditions such as herpes can flare up when the body is weak. Links have also been made between stress and asthma, eczema, and diabetes.

Some studies have found a relationship between long-term stress and heart disease. But many other factors contribute to heart disease and one study found that people with stressful jobs suffered no more heart attacks than those doing less pressured work.

Signs of stress

If you recognize that you are regularly suffering from two of the following symptoms, then the likelihood is that you are feeling stressed or overwrought and need to look at how to make changes in your work and home life. You will need to take steps to reduce your stress, to concentrate on improving your health, and to relax more. The symptoms are:

• Anxiety and panic attacks.
• Insomnia and sleep problems.
• High blood pressure.
• Heart palpitations.
• Headaches, indigestion, or breathlessness.
• Aggressive behavior.
• Drinking too much alcohol or taking drugs to calm yourself down.
• Experiencing a lack of sex drive or becoming obsessive about sex.
• Suffering aches and pains in the neck, shoulders, arms, and legs.
• Stomachache or cramps.
• Eye strain or migraines.
• Lack of appetite.
• Fainting spells.
• Tendency to sweat for no reason.
• Lack of appetite or unusual craving for food.

Tips to relieve stress

There are several methods that you can use to reduce the symptoms of stress:

● Close your eyes briefly to encourage relaxing brain waves.

● Slowly take three deep breaths, breathing in from your abdomen.

● Drink a cup of warm tea to relax you, or try an herbal tea.

● Have a good yawn; it helps to stretch and relax your face muscles.

Life today is a constant struggle. Stress comes from worrying about the mortgage, meeting tight deadlines, or having arguments at home. Even ordinary household tasks, driving, and planning a holiday can affect us. But don't resort to alcohol or drugs—just learn how to relax more.

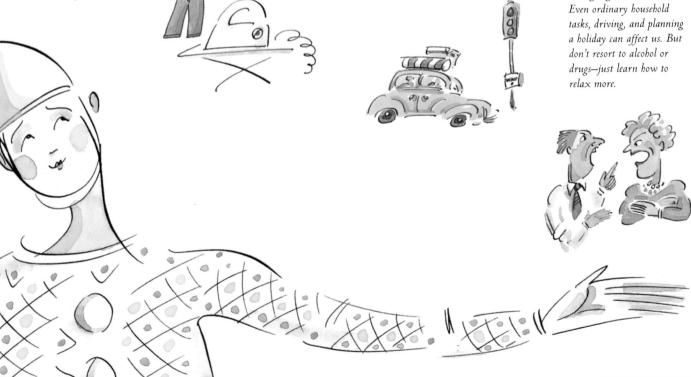

Crisis Management

Everyone at some point in their lives must confront times of crisis—crunch times when their life is irreversibly changed. Bereavement, divorce, loss of a job or a home, or a serious illness can all trigger a state of crisis from which it seems impossible to recover. Sometimes one stressful event occurs that you manage to cope with, only for you to be knocked down by another serious event happening at the same time. It could be that you move into a new house the same week you separate from a long-term partner, or your child gets very ill at the same time your partner becomes unemployed.

We all have our own unique level of coping before the cracks begin to show. Negative or challenging life events can put excessive pressure on people, but it usually takes two or more negative events to set a personal crisis in motion. It can sometimes be a good event combined with a personal loss that tips the scales. You could be informed of a job promotion with increased responsibilities at the same time as getting the news of the death of a parent. But, whatever the causes, it is important not to deny to yourself or to your family and close friends that you are suffering. A crisis can make a big impact on your mental and physical health and it needs to be dealt with so that your body and mind can be given a chance to adjust to the circumstances and you can start the healing process.

In today's insecure world, a growing problem is the incredible demands that are being made of people in the workplace. Often people are expected to achieve unrealistically high goals and work excessive hours to do so. This can adversely affect their self-confidence and their sense of personal well-being and security. When subjected to high levels of work stress, people need to recognize when they can no longer cope and discuss the situation with their bosses or partner—or seek professional help if they feel they can't resolve the pressures themselves.

Sometimes a minicrisis can be resolved after a few days of reflection and a confidential talk with a friend who listens well and whose opinions you value. By talking things through, you can often put your problems into perspective and identify new ways of sorting them out, perhaps by dealing with a problem bit by bit rather than all at once. But at other times, professional help may well be necessary to guide you through a dark, tumultuous time.

Facing a personal crisis

A crisis could be a difficult situation that you might have to deal with in the world at large or it might involve an acute personal or psychological problem. Whatever the cause, it is important to remember that a crisis can be a turning point as well as a distressing time of emotional difficulty.

Often a crisis can be brought on by trying to live up to the expectations of others at the expense of your own needs. Thus a crisis is perhaps a time to think about what you want to do rather than what you ought to do to please other people or to meet society's expectations. A difficult time could be the launching point for a more fulfilling life.

Remember that problems can be shared, so it is a good idea to talk about them. Friends and family are a good starting point and often your family physician or HMO, who have access to many resources and contacts, can help. You may also want to join a support group geared to your individual problem.

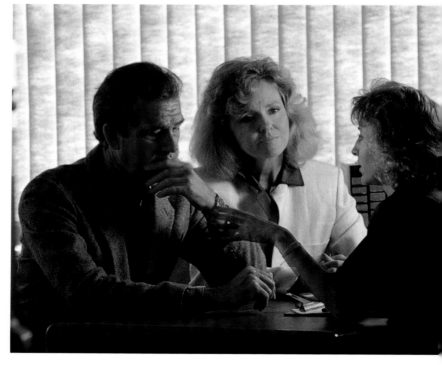

The Stress Scale

In the 1970s a scale was published in the *Journal of Psychosomatic Research*. It detailed 43 common life events that were potentially harmful to everyone's health and happiness The scale was drawn up by two American doctors, T. H. Holme and R. H. Rahe. The impact of these 43 life events is measured on a scale of 1 to 100. Research showed that if a person accumulates a score of more than 300 in one year, there is an 80 percent risk of sickness during the next two years. A score between 150 and 300 gives a 50 percent risk of sickness during the same period. But what has to be remembered is that it is a person's reaction to an event that causes the level of stress. A child leaving home, for example, for a possessive mother could feel like 100 points, while to another mother who had dealt with a troublesome teenager, it might seem more like 10 points. The top 30 most threatening events are listed below:

	Scale		Scale
Death of spouse or partner	100	Change of financial status	39
Divorce	73	Death of friend	37
Marital separation	65	Change in line of work	36
Jail sentence or being institutionalized	63	Change in number of marital arguments	35
Death of close member of family	63	Large mortgage taken out	31
Illness or injury	53	Mortgage or loan foreclosed	30
Marriage	50	Responsibility change	29
Loss of job	47	Child leaves home	29
Reconciliation with marriage partner	45	In-law problems	29
Retirement	45	Personal achievement realized	28
Health problem of close member of family	44	Wife starts or stops work	26
Pregnancy	40	Starting at new school	26
Sex problems	39	Leaving school	26
Addition to family	39	Change in living conditions	25
Major change at work	39	Change in personal habits	24

The benefits of counseling

Sometimes when you are in a crisis situation, no matter how you try to help yourself through it, you can feel you are sinking and realize that you can no longer cope on your own. It is at the point when you feel there is no way out that you should seek help from a professional counselor or therapist who is trained to help you through these very difficult times.

It takes real inner strength and courage to recognize the severity of your problems and admit to yourself that you need help, but once you have made the move you won't look back. You will be able to talk through your fears and frustrations with the counselor, who will help you build up your confidence again and discuss ways of restructuring and rebuilding your life in a much more positive way. If your crisis is the result of a partner dying, for example, your local bereavement counselor might well be the lifeline that you need to help you come to terms with your new life on your own.

You can share your grief, anger, and despair with the therapist, who understands what you are going through. You can tell him or her your darkest, unhappiest thoughts and also explore various strategies that will help you cope better, little by little and from day to day.

You might want to consider joining a bereavement support group if you need to discuss your feelings and experiences with other people who are also going through a similar experience.

If you or your partner have suffered a series of events that have made you reach a crisis point in your life, talking through the problems with a trained counselor can help you to come to terms with them and to cope again.

If you are with a friend or colleague when they receive bad news they may show signs of shock. There are things you can do to help:

• If they feel faint, sit them on a chair and place their head between their knees. Otherwise just have them sit quietly.

• Make sure they don't forget to breathe. Guide them to breathe in and out from the abdomen.

• If they start to hyperventilate, get them to breathe deeply into a paper bag.

• Keep them warm by covering them with a coat or blanket.

• Gently rub the shocked person's hands, feet, or upper back to try to calm them.

• If the shocked person's condition worsens, get medical help right away.

Positive Thinking

Positive thinking is the key to everything you do in your life. Your work, your relationships, and your feelings about yourself will all be greatly improved just by developing a more positive attitude. The techniques that are described here are powerful and successful enough to be used by psychologists to help people who are suffering from serious depression, but you can also use them to make your own life fuller and much more rewarding.

"Look on the bright side" can be one of the most irritating pieces of advice that is given. You can be in a bad mood, expounding on how impossible things are at work, or how no one at home is helping you, and all your so-called friend can suggest is that you take a more optimistic view of things. Actually, your friend's advice is well worth taking; but the difficulty most people have is that they don't know how to look on the bright side. What's more, they can't see how it would make any difference to their everyday lives.

But thinking positively can make an enormous difference in what you do and what you can achieve. When you speak very negatively to friends you are saying that you don't feel in control. And you are not. You can't stop problems from happening at work or at home—but there is one thing you can control: How you think about your life and how you react to different situations. The way you think about what is happening to you affects the way you behave.

For example, if you project the attitude that the world is a hostile place and most people are against you, you are going to behave in a suspicious and defensive way. People will respond to you in an unfriendly and hostile manner, which will prove that you were right to distrust the world in the first place. Or will it? Doesn't it just show that the manner in which you approach events affects what happens to you?

Neurologists now know that people's eyes do not work like cameras, passively recording whatever they see, but that instead they are "virtual reality" studios. The brain actually constructs the view of the world from the limited amount of information that the human senses select. Therefore, the brain can be equally creative with what happens to you.

That doesn't mean to say that you can dismiss the impact on people of the death of a close family member, personal disease, failure of a marriage or long-term relationship, or major disappointments, but it does mean that there is always more than one way of seeing things.

Even when you are at your most depressed and there seems no way out of your circumstances, if you try to see some positive aspects of the situation you're in, however minor, you will start to feel better, the future will seem brighter, and you will be more confident in yourself.

Negative thinking

These are some of the negative thoughts that you can have about your life when you have gotten into a depressed way of thinking. The way to deal with them is to notice what you are doing and then start to challenge them because they are never the whole truth.

• Overdramatizing–always predicting the worst: "Nobody will want me;" "I'll never work again."
• Overgeneralizing–because something unfortunate happened once it will always happen: "I always make a mess of things. I can never do it."
• Exaggerating–making negative events more important than they should be: "This is the end. I'll never do it."
• Ignoring the positive–when something good happens you play it down or ignore it saying: "It was just luck;" "This old thing? It's just a hand-me-down."
• Mind-reading–assuming you know what others are thinking: "They don't want me."

Positive thoughts

Once you have spotted when your unhelpful thinking patterns and depressing thoughts start, you are more than halfway toward changing them. Now you can make a positive diary. Look at the negative thoughts that you accepted so unquestioningly, and start to challenge them, highlighting your strengths. You can learn to identify your skills, attributes, and talents; you might say: "It's true I'm alone at the moment, but I've made good relationships in the past and I will again;" "The job is hard but the people are nice."

Then you should begin to counter some examples of negative thinking by saying: "It's not true I'm not good at anything. I organized the Christmas party brilliantly;" "I sometimes make mistakes but most of the time I don't." You are not looking for a right way of seeing things, just one that makes you feel better and gives you more possibilities.

Soon you won't need to make a diary. You'll be able to catch yourself thinking negatively and the fact that you have recognized the pattern will more than likely make you laugh—and you'll instantly feel better and more positive about everything.

The negative spiral

Most of us are very familiar with the way our thoughts affect our feelings. If we listen to sad music, we become melancholy and our thoughts, too, become sad. In the same way, we are expert at thinking negative thoughts about ourselves and allowing them to take control. If we let them remain in control for long enough, we become depressed. Such depressed thoughts can be very strong during times of intense personal pressure and pain. All we can think about is dejection, defeat, and despair. When the stress is severe, particularly when rejection is involved, we are especially vulnerable to negative suggestion. To see any positives during difficult times can seem pointless, but positive thinking can give you a way of stepping back from your current situation and reviewing other ways of handling it. To make yourself switch from a negative to positive attitude is an essential skill to be learned for your own happiness and to control stress successfully.

Try keeping a negative diary. For a few days just write down your negative feelings and summarize your thoughts. It might read something like: "Sad . . . I shouldn't have taken this job;" "Depressed . . . I'm all on my own," and so on. This will help you put your moods into a clearer perspective.

When you do the visualization exercise, choose three positive images from your past life to make you feel optimistic.

Creative visualization exercise

The most powerful way of thinking positively is to use visualization techniques. When problems overwhelm you or you just need to be positive, practice this short "Circles of Excellence" exercise:

• Shut your eyes and put yourself in a positive state–then pick a phrase that represents it, such as, "I can achieve." Then imagine a circle on the floor. Fill it in with a strong, bright color, then associate this color with praise.
• Next, remember a time when you were optimistic and imagine it is happening in that circle. When the memory and the colors fill the circle, say your phrase and step forward to join it.
• Then imagine a second circle; fill it with another color, recalling another optimistic time. Say your phrase, hold on to the first feeling, and step forward and merge with the second. Do it a third time; your anger will vanish and you'll feel confident and happy.

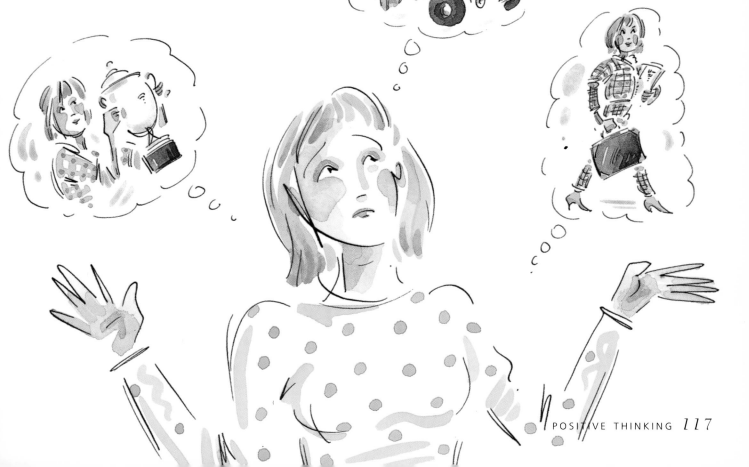

Personal Happiness

A major problem for most of us is that we don't really know how to enjoy ourselves. On a physical level we have a greater choice of food, clothes, and entertainment than any other society in history. However, it does not seem to make us very happy. At least half the population will have a problem at some time in their lives that will make them drink too much or resort to tranquilizers. Most often, these problems are a sure sign of something wrong at a deeper level—perhaps mental depression or a lack of self-esteem.

But happiness is essential to our general well-being. In fact, some research done in this country shows that enjoying ourselves is good for us. People who report being happy in their day-to-day lives have lower levels of stress and are less likely to suffer heart attacks.

That old adage about money not bringing happiness is true, because happiness does not depend on events, but on how we interpret them. One of the more surprising findings of psychological research is that one year after winning big in a lottery, winners rate themselves as being no more happy than they were before. This is because the way we determine our measure of happiness is by comparing the way we feel now with how we expected to feel.

Research has found that the way physical pleasures work best for us is in frequent small doses. One recent study asked several hundred people to report every few hours for six weeks on how happy they were feeling. Those who constantly took pleasure in the little things in life—the smell of freshly baked bread, the look of a beautiful flower, a tune on the radio, or a friend laughing—were the ones who described themselves as the most happy.

Relationships

Relationships can cause the greatest highs and the lowest lows in your life. Creating loving relationships is vital to human beings. Each of us responds in a different way to the need to harmonize and to feel complete and whole. Getting intimate relationships sorted out is probably the single most effective way of improving the quality of your life. It is certainly good for your health—the pain of losing your love in a long-term relationship can actually damage your immune system. People need to learn to communicate honestly with each other and give each other consideration and commitment.

Yet all too often we give up on relationships. The divorce rate is one in three marriages and rising. Almost all of us have a number of angry, sad, or unhappy relationships to look back on. But you can make your current relationship a lot better.

Relationships should be fun and fulfilling, but to stay that way they need care and attention. If you seriously want to improve the way you get along with your partner there are three things to consider:

• Each of us can change only ourselves—we often have a long list of our partner's faults, but only *they* can make changes or be more understanding.
• Change can be slow—people often want a relationship to stay the same even when it doesn't work very well. Making changes needs courage and persistence.
• Set a time limit—some relationships need more work than others. If you've made changes and you still wish the other person were different, think about marital counseling *(opposite)*.

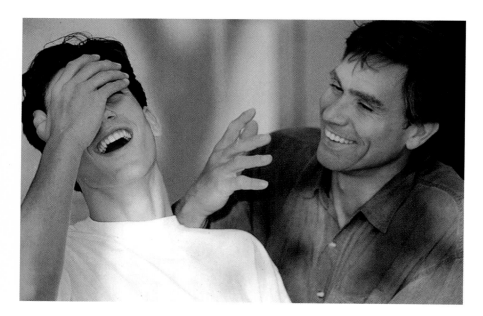

Pleasure can be gained from so many aspects of our lives. Telling a friend or your child an amusing anecdote or story that makes them laugh can make both of you feel good.

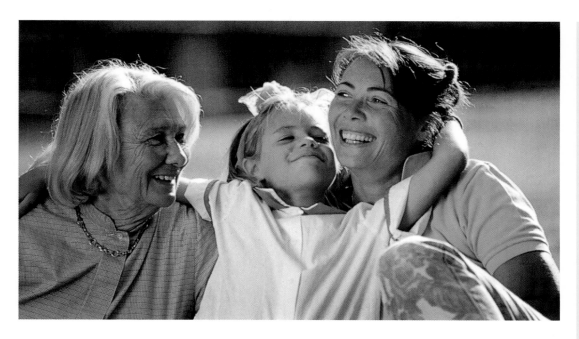

Social pleasures

Human beings are very social animals, so just keeping a positive outlook and balancing stimulation with relaxation is not enough. We have evolved to have strong relationships with those around us, starting with parents and caregivers and maturing to lovers and friends.

Research shows that people who can form close and loving partnerships report being happier and staying healthier. But the benefits of a good relationship do not stop with a couple. Keeping in touch with relatives, having plenty of friends, and being on good terms with the neighbors are also linked to well-being. People who are involved in their community are two-and-a-half times less likely to suffer from heart attacks.

When it comes to having a good network of friends, women tend to keep in touch more than men, which may be why health statistics show that older married men are healthier than older single men. Health advice for men tends to concentrate on exercise and diet, but learning how to have close friendships might prove to be just as important to longevity.

Having a warm, loving relationship with your family and close friends can make you feel happy, and can help you to stay well.

Marital counseling

Sooner or later many relationships reach a point where at least one of you feels you can't go on—maybe because one of you has had an affair or the fights are too nasty, or one wants to change and the other doesn't. If there are also strong reasons for staying together, these are the times when counseling can help. Research shows there is a much better chance of saving a relationship with counseling if couples go *before* they reach the breaking point.

Marriage counseling can provide you with neutral ground where the two of you can discuss the issues, or even yell and scream them at each other. The difference is that you are doing it with a trained therapist who can act as a neutral party. His or her job is to help you sort out the real issues and allow a solution to emerge.

This may involve uncovering deep, unspoken feelings. Quite possibly there will be surprises—"I never knew you felt like that" will often be a common reaction. After a few sessions you should at least have some new skills to help you communicate better. When you have made it clear what both of you want and what each is prepared to give, then you can make a reasonable decision on whether to rebuild the relationship or to part.

Tips for being happy every day

To get the most out of life, happiness is an essential element. Think about what makes you happy and try some of the tips below:

● Laugh as often as you can. It stimulates the pleasure centers and can increase your heart rate.

● Notice what activities give you pleasure: Is it challenging ones, such as play acting, or is it relaxing ones like yoga?

● Make physical contact often with friends, children, and lovers: It stimulates the relaxation centers in the brain.

● Take it easy. A steady half-hour walk will lift your mood and make you feel more relaxed and happy.

● Do something for someone else—doing a good turn or helping someone can give you great pleasure.

● Have fun on your own watching some old comedy videos.

Self-Acceptance

Everybody knows that self-confidence is a strong factor behind success and most people have a friend or acquaintance who seems to possess this mysterious but vital quality. They seem to sail through difficult situations, achieve the impossible on difficult projects, or walk away unscathed when things don't work out. But how do they do it? What is the essence of believing in yourself?

So many people seem to lack confidence and constantly run themselves down. Sometimes it may seem as though you have never been confident. In fact, that is almost certainly not true. Self-confidence is a skill that can be learned. Some people are better at it than others but anyone can learn it. Everybody feels confident about the things they do well.

Psychologists' questionnaires reveal that almost no one is confident all the time. If you ask apparently confident people how they feel they will often say something like: "I feel great giving a party, but ask me to stand up and sing and I go to pieces."

Everybody has different areas of confidence and the best way to increase the number of them is simply to pretend. Studies show that if you pretend to be confident it works almost as well as the real thing. If you demonstrate confidence people are going to believe in you, and having people believe in you is one of the greatest boosts to your confidence. So pretending to be confident can actually make you confident for real.

So how do you start to increase your confidence? First of all you need to notice the times when you feel self-assured. Once you become aware of what being confident feels like, you will have something to build on.

Select the areas that you need to feel confident in: Being confident, for example, about public speaking when you work in a library is not a top priority, but you do need to be able to deal effectively with people.

Get a sense of what it is about all those different situations that makes you feel so anxious. If it is that you don't feel you're worth very much, try saying some affirmations (*opposite*) over and over to yourself.

Try to visualize yourself in a situation where you need to be confident. Imagine you need to give an interesting talk about work or a hobby, for example, and see yourself being confident throughout the speech and notice how accomplished you look and how good you feel.

You need to set yourself some goals. Start first with easy ones. If you find talking to your boss is a problem, try approaching a less senior figure at work and give him or her your viewpoints on current problems. Focus the conversation on a topic that you know well and feel comfortable talking about.

Try to use some relaxation techniques as part of your confidence-building practice. Breathe deeply two or three times from your abdomen to calm you.

If you are going through a period in your life when you are very unsure of yourself, regularly try to say a positive self-affirmation while looking at yourself in a mirror. You will soon start to feel better and really believe in what you are saying.

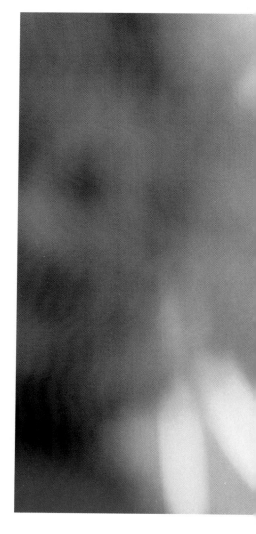

Give yourself treats

When you are trying to learn anything new, rewards work much better than criticism and blame. Your confidence-building exercises will go even better if you reward yourself with a treat afterward. Don't treat yourself with something that is going to annoy others–for example, don't buy flowers if it gives your partner hay fever–or something that might trigger your own guilt, such as chocolates, if you know that you will eat them all at once.

Most of your treats should be small, quick, and frequent. Depending on your preferences they might be:

Physical:
- Go for a pleasant walk.
- Stay in bed an extra hour.
- Treat yourself to some new clothes.
- Take some singing lessons.

Mental:
- Read a good novel.
- Go out to a movie with a friend.
- Listen to your favorite music.

Spiritual:
- Have some time alone.
- Meditate to calm and refresh your mind.
- Allow some time to do yoga.

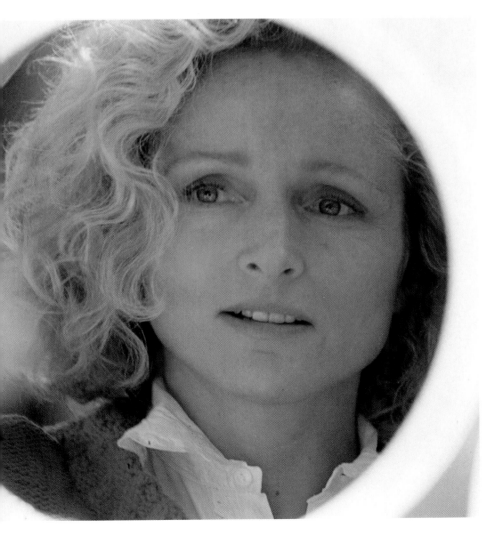

Affirmations

To increase your confidence and to help change aspects of your personality that you don't like, you need to love and to make friends with yourself. This can be difficult, but affirmations can help you do it. You have got to really believe in what you're saying, though, or it won't work.

- Look in the mirror and say: "I love you." If you really say it with positive meaning you'll be amazed how you can come to believe it.
- If you feel that you can't cope, say: "I'm strong and capable and can achieve everything I attempt." Soon the belief will be instilled in you and you will cope.
- When you are feeling tense and strung out, repeat to yourself: "I am relaxed." Visualize looking relaxed and feeling calm and you will soon feel the benefits.
- If you feel you always fail at whatever you attempt, keep repeating to yourself: "I'm a success." Soon you will be achieving your objectives.
- When work is getting you down, tell yourself: "I will resolve the problems." If you really believe in this, before long you will find solutions.
- Don't keep criticizing your figure; look at yourself and say: "I have a great body." Soon you will stop criticizing your body's inadequacies and emphasize what is good about it.
- If you are forever calling yourself stupid, turn it around and say: "I'm smart, intelligent, and wise," and forget your self-criticism.
- If you fear that you appear hard and cold, say to yourself: "I'm a wonderful, warm, and loving person." If you really believe in what you are saying, a genuine warmth will come through.
- Emphasize your positive qualities. Try saying: "I'm attractive, loved, and bring warmth and comfort to the ones I love."
- Try saying: "We're going to be all right," when you seem to be facing financial difficulties. They won't go away but you will feel more able to cope with your financial problems.

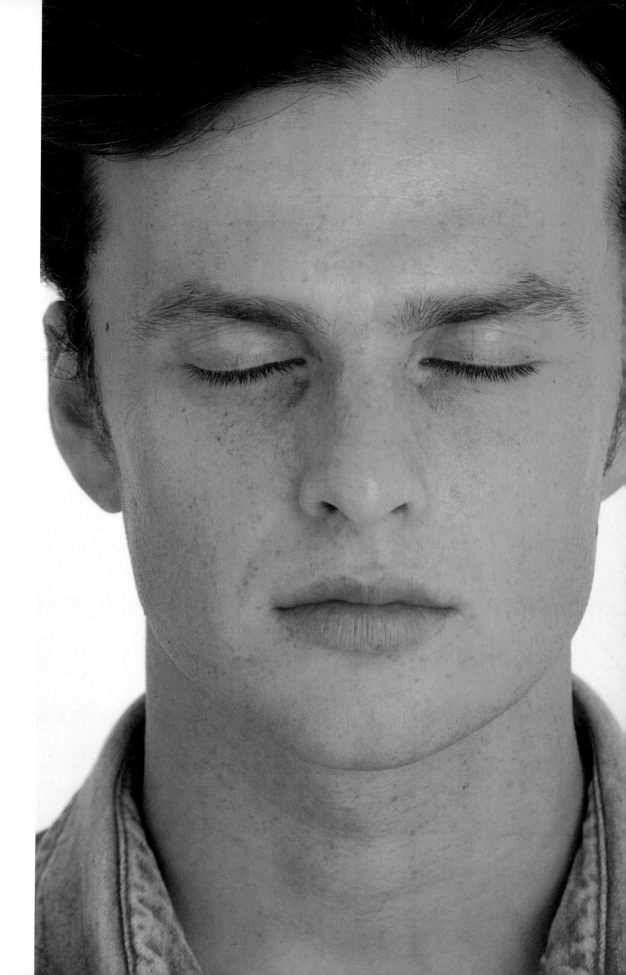

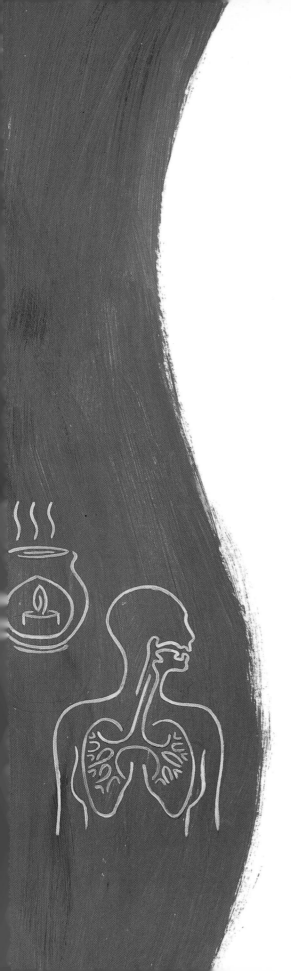

7
Mind-Body Relaxation

The importance of relaxation in our busy lives cannot be over-emphasized. Life today finds more people than ever facing increasing demands at work, new responsibilities and challenges, insecurities, and a whole mixture of stressful situations. Now more than ever we need to take regular breaks from work and make some time for ourselves.

One of the ways we can help ourselves is to learn some relaxation techniques: Both deep breathing and meditation, for example, can really help to calm our bodies and improve our general health.

We all need to make some leisure time to counteract the stresses of our complex lifestyles and to restore our well-being. We need to enjoy some quality time with our partners, children, and friends and maybe take up a hobby or pastime that is stimulating and gives us pleasure. Try not to think too much about the future; appreciate the here and now.

Breathing Techniques

In the Western world most of us take breathing and our entire respiratory system for granted. The extraordinary difference between East and West is that in India and China, for example, the emphasis on breathing properly to achieve good health and a true state of well-being is immense. Here in the West we only consider our lungs and the whole subject of breathing when we are fighting for air because of pollution, pollen, or a degenerative lung disease. Because we are not taught proper breathing techniques, many people develop bad habits out of ignorance, combined with laziness. We breathe too fast, or shallow breathe, and retain too much stale air in our lungs because we begin to breathe in again before we have finished breathing out.

If you are feeling tense or are suffering from stress, you can breathe too shallowly and can possibly start to hyperventilate. If you are breathing in a stressed manner you can become mentally disorientated and emotionally uncertain. To breathe correctly you must use your nose and not your mouth. The nose is designed to cleanse and warm the air before it reaches your lungs. Relaxed breathing is a natural breathing method that involves deep, long, regular breaths. This type of breathing gives the balance and poise necessary for maintaining the equilibrium of both the mind and body.

Learning how to breathe properly is an important part of everyone's education. The increasing popularity of Indian yoga in the West is largely due to the practical and clear health teachings of pranayama, the art of the science of breathing, which is practiced alongside yoga.

The breath of life

Whole healthy breathing is taught in various cultures. In India and China especially, the respiratory system is considered to have an important part to play in preventing illness. The Hindu word "prana" means "breath of life." More than just the breath, prana refers to an energy that supports and energizes all life; Hindus believe that these elements are contained in the air we breathe. When we breathe in, we then also breathe in these special powers.

Pranayama is the ancient science and art of breath control and regulation. It is not just control of the respiration; it is the deliberate direction of prana throughout the body that matters. Yogis instruct their students always to breathe through the nose when possible–the mouth is for eating, talking, and kissing!

Pranayama consists of three types of breath control: inhalation (puraka), exhalation (recaka), and retention (kumbhaka). You can learn to use your breath properly by going to any good yoga class.

Chi kung is the Chinese equivalent of India's pranayama. Chi kung also means energy and breathing control, and it has been a formal branch of Chinese medicine for more than 2,000 years. In China it is regarded as a science. Practitioners of Chi kung, in both the East and the West, believe that the body's supply of vital energy is created by correct breathing and that practicing this technique is the essential key to promoting our well-being and longevity.

"You can live two months without food and two weeks without water, but you can only live a few minutes without air."
HUNG YI-HSIANG, TAOIST MASTER

Complete yoga breathing

Sit comfortably, either in a chair, cross-legged on a mat (right), or on your heels (below). Keep your spine straight. Close your eyes, concentrate on your navel and center yourself on this area. Breathe out and then in through the nose, expanding first the abdomen, then the ribs, chest, and collarbone as you count to eight. Then exhale through the nose, contracting the abdomen, ribs, and chest, and finally lowering the collarbone and shoulders to the count of eight. Repeat three to six times at the beginner's stage. This exercise helps to calm the nervous system, oxygenates the blood, and also increases lung capacity.

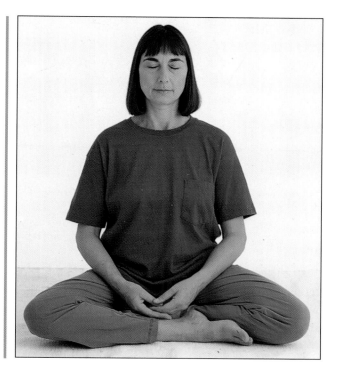

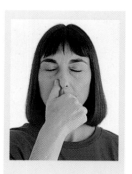

One-nostril breathing

Close the right nostril with the right thumb. Slowly inhale deeply through the left nostril and then exhale. Do this three to six times, then repeat on other side. This calms the mind and balances energy.

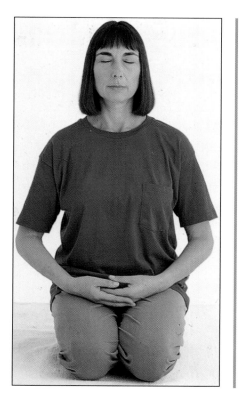

Kumbhaka (retention) breathing

This exercise can be done sitting, standing, or lying down. It is the same as the first exercise but you focus on your heart and extend your breath by holding it to the count of four after inhalation and before you begin exhalation (left). Always breathe in and out to the count of eight; you can slowly hold your breath longer, but don't strain and don't do the exercise if you have a heart condition. This calms the nervous system.

Ujjayi (sitting or lying down) breathing

Sit, stand, or lie down and focus on your throat area (right). Exhale and then inhale through your nose, counting to eight as in the first exercise. Hold your breath for eight seconds and exhale making a long drawn-out "S" sound, but count to 16. Do the exercise three times. This breathing stimulates the endocrine glands and is good for low blood pressure.

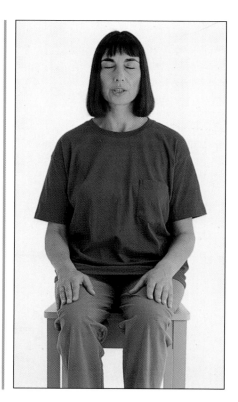

Meditation

Transcendental meditation

This type of meditation, also known as TM, has become one of the most popular and widely known meditation systems in the Western world over the last 30 years. It was introduced by the Maharishi Mahesh Yogi to the Beatles in India during the 1960s, and it has attracted a large following over the three decades since. It appeals to many people, not only those interested in holistic therapies but business people, who learn TM to control their stress levels and promote a sense of well-being in their personal and professional lives.

In his book *Ageless Body, Timeless Mind* Deepak Chopra says: "TM is based on the silent repetition of a specific Sanskrit word, or mantra, whose sound vibrations gradually lead the mind out of its normal thinking process and into the silence that underlies thought. As such, a mantra is a very specific message inserted into the nervous system."

The purpose of meditation is to let go of all the normal thoughts and worries of the material world, freeing the mind to experience the peace of the spiritual world.

To learn the Transcendental Meditation technique properly you should receive instruction from a trained TM teacher.

In the Hindu religion mandalas are often made from flowers for festivals or other occasions. The patterns of concentric circles direct the believer toward the center to use this point for meditation.

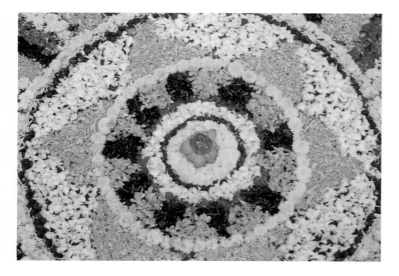

The mind is a vast, mostly uncharted territory in which few of us ever travel more than a tiny distance: What we call living in normal consciousness could be likened to living on the fringe of an immense, undiscovered land. Just think how busy our minds are during waking hours. They are usually in a state of constant thought: making endless plans, speculating about problems, reliving memories, mulling over worries, and processing all the things needed to be done in that day. It is not often that you stop this never-ending flow of thought and try to experience more of an inner peace.

Meditation is a process of stilling the mind and developing a completely calm mental state. It is a simple form of mental relaxation where the mind is emptied of its thoughts in favor of one thought, image, or word that is concentrated on.

Eddie and Debbie Shapiro, meditation teachers and holistic healers, describe it as follows: "Throughout the ages, meditation has been used to enter within and explore the wonders that are there. True meditation is a fully conscious natural awareness, a mind that is clear and free. Through relaxation and meditation we unfold the vast inner world that lies hidden at the core of our being.

"When we practice sitting or walking meditation, allowing the mind to become quiet, receptive, and still, we have the opportunity to go beyond the normal chatter that fills our days and creates all the chaos and fear in our minds. When you meditate you make or allow time to connect with the essence of life, to find the *self* beyond the ego. Here you can develop an inner awareness of the mind as it really is, beneath the superficiality."

The practice of meditation is usually associated with Eastern religions or philosophies such as Buddhism, Hinduism, Zen and Tao, and yoga, but it is also very much a part of the Judeo-Christian tradition.

In Buddhism and Hinduism an image is often focused on to aid the meditative process. One of these images is a mandala—a picture that is normally circular, symbolizing the universe. Alternately, a mantra—a sacred word or syllable—is spoken repetitively to concentrate the mind and to get the person meditating in tune with their inner selves. Both these techniques are now widely used by people in the Western world who employ the meditation process regularly.

"Meditation is not a means to an end. It is both the means and the end."
J. KRISHNAMURTI

Meditation is recognized not only as a powerful tool for personal growth but also as a therapeutic process that helps to combat stress and prevent stress-related illnesses, from high blood pressure and asthma to cancer and heart disease. It is an effective way of relieving pain, of helping to alleviate chronic back problems, and of enhancing the immune system. It can even help to treat people suffering from the HIV infection and AIDS. Meditation has become a way of life for millions of Westerners in recent decades as the reputation of its life-affirming qualities has become firmly established and proven.

Chanting

Chanting, or Mantra Yoga, is the process of prayer and invocation. The sound vibrations of certain mantras stimulate a very powerful, constructive, and harmonizing effect on the mind and body. Chanting mantras–like the sounds Aum, Om, Ra, Ma, and Ram–focuses the restless mind on a certain vibratory pattern, eliminating distraction and enabling the mind to become more still and meditative. Chanting is also good for the body because it naturally exercises your respiratory system and therefore promotes oxygenation and circulation, and helps to eliminate waste.

In *Ageless Body, Timeless Mind*, Deepak Chopra discusses how meditation, using mantras or images, helps to lower biological age. He says: "The connection between aging and stress hormones has been strongly demonstrated, but the problem of how to control these hormones remains. Because the stress reaction can be triggered in a split second and without warning, it is impossible for us to control the molecules themselves. However, there is one mind-body technique that goes directly to the root of the stress response by releasing the remembered stresses that trigger new stress: meditation. Levels of cortisol and adrenalin are often found to be lower in long-term meditators, and their coping mechanisms almost always tend to be stronger than average."

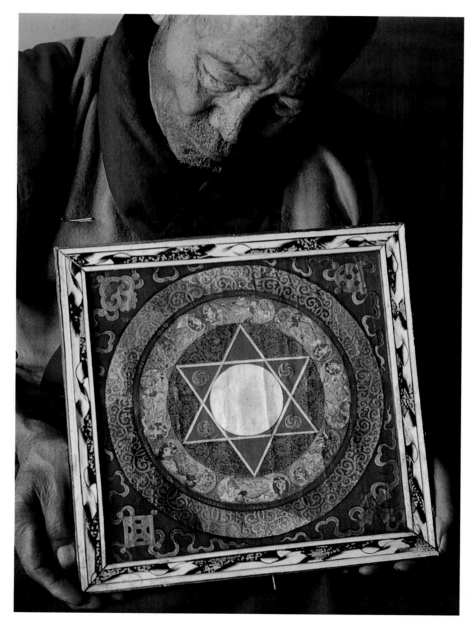

Here a Tibetan Buddhist monk is holding a mandala (an image used for meditating). The middle of the star in the center of the picture is the energy point for people to focus on when meditating. The geometry of a mandala represents a being in harmony with the outside universe.

The meditating technique

Sitting still and doing nothing is the only way to give your mind a complete rest. Even while asleep, the body may be resting and recovering its vitality, but the mind is entangled in dreams, which can be so mentally exhausting that we sometimes wake up less rested than before we went to sleep. But before you can learn to meditate you must acquire the art of being still. You may be surprised to discover just how difficult that is, so do not be alarmed if it is hard to achieve at first. With patience and practice you will learn how to meditate.

When learning how to sit still and do nothing, beginners should bear in mind a few basics. The major points of attention are stated in an ancient text: "Shut off the three external treasures of hearing, sight, and speech in order to cultivate the three internal treasures of essence, energy, and spirit." At first you may find steadying the mind difficult enough, let alone stilling it. Do not worry. Everyone experiences the "playful monkey of the mind" and the frustration that goes with it. The next thing you must develop after relaxation and steady, natural breathing is patience. This quality more than any other will help you learn to meditate.

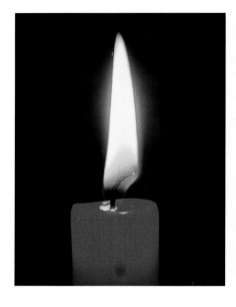

A very useful meditation technique is to concentrate and soften your gaze on an "outer," or external object such as a candle flame. Concentrating your mind on a single object will help you focus and empty your mind of all its thoughts. This will then allow you to develop your powers of relaxation, concentration, and oneness.

The art of meditation

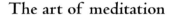

1. Find a comfortable space
The first thing you must do to prepare for meditation is find a quiet place where you feel the atmosphere and conditions are conducive to a retreat from the reality around you. Even if in the beginning you only meditate for 5 to10 minutes, building up to about 20, it is important to find a spot where nothing will interfere with your mental exercises.

After you have learned to meditate, you will be more adept at shutting out the distractions around you and you will even be able to meditate in motion, for example, while walking along a country lane or strolling in a park.

2. Find a comfortable position
After finding your space, you must find the posture that is appropriate and comfortable for your meditation. It is not necessary to sit in the lotus position or cross-legged on the floor to meditate. You can meditate anywhere you feel comfortable, even sitting on a chair.

3. Check your posture
Your back should be relaxed, upright, controlled, and erect but *without* being fixed and rigid. This upright posture will help you to maintain your concentration and steady your mind. One way to help you

find and hold this posture is to imagine a string gently pulling you up through the crown of your head, as described in the Alexander Technique *(page 80)*.

4. Relax muscles and organs
To help you focus the mind, release and relax all your muscles and internal organs by autosuggestion. Some people like to instruct themselves to release and relax by going through the entire body from the top of the head to the tips of the toes.

5. Practice breathing
To help slow down the mind, steady your breath naturally by taking a deep, flowing, and gentle breath. Allow it to emerge without force and without judgment. By doing a relaxation exercise first, you should have little or no problem finding your lowered respiratory rate reflected in slower, deeper breathing. They go together–for relaxation to occur the breath must become steady so you will naturally acquire a slow, even, flowing breath that reflects your inner state.

6. Follow your breath
Follow your breath as you inhale and exhale. Some people find this a very effective, simple, first meditation exercise. Just meditate on your breath, following it

on its journey in and out of the body. Be aware of your breath. Notice its unique qualities and the way it ebbs and flows from your body. Observe your breath without judgment and without suggestion. Just observe.

7. Remain on the plateau
Allow yourself to remain in this state of deep tranquillity. Enjoy the freedom from worldly cares. When you feel adequately refreshed you may stop. Many people worry about losing themselves in meditation, as if it were a form of self-hypnosis that they cannot control. That is not meditation. While meditating you may not be part of what is going on around you but you will always be able to rejoin the world when you wish.

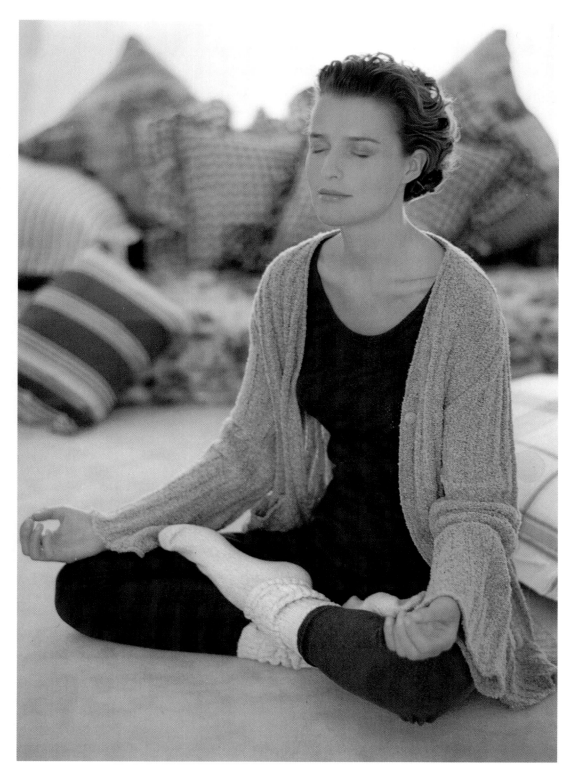

Meditation can be done anywhere, at any time, and in any position—even on a beach—provided your back is upright. You do not need to be able to sit cross-legged or in the lotus position. All you need is to choose a quiet place where you feel comfortable and shut off from the outside world and you can relax.

Rest and Sleep

Rest is what keeps our bodies going, but all too often we seem to neglect it, rushing through our lives as though we expect there to be 28 hours of the day, rather than 24. If we don't allow adequate time for rest and sleep we can literally run our bodies down, making ourselves vulnerable to illness.

Rest needs to be planned into our lives. Regular vacations are also important, as are short breaks, to rediscover our partners and to appreciate our children away from the hurly-burly of life at home.

Sleep is also essential to our lives. In fact, we spend about a third of our lives asleep, but it is still a mystery exactly why. We certainly can't do without sleep. In 1959 disc jockey Peter Tripp stayed awake for 200 hours for charity. Toward the end he couldn't concentrate at all and was having hallucinations—a tweed suit seemed like a mat of furry worms. Depriving rats of sleep for a month will kill them, but not before some intriguing contradictions occur—they simultaneously eat ravenously and lose massive amounts of weight.

Some researchers believe that sleep developed because we couldn't hunt in the dark; it made sense to save energy at night. Instead, couples could have sex, ensuring the reproduction of the species, and rest, allowing their bodies to prepare for daylight activity. This is a version of the common-sense view that says we sleep to rest and refresh ourselves, but scientists have found that for part of the night our brains do not rest. By recording the brain activity of sleeping people, they have found two periods of sleep: orthodox and paradoxical, which alternate in 90-minute cycles.

After falling asleep we go into orthodox mode, when the body takes it easy. The blood pressure drops, heart and breathing rates slow down, and oxygen consumption is at its lowest. This lasts for an hour or so until paradoxical sleep takes over.

This latter type of sleep is the time when we dream, which paradoxically uses up any energy saved in the previous period. The brain becomes almost as active as when it is awake, although the balance of brain chemicals is different and blood in the brain flows faster. The eyes can be seen moving under their lids, but the sleeper cannot move; most muscles are deeply relaxed and reflexes are lost.

People vary enormously in how much sleep they need. For some, three hours is fine, others swear they cannot do with less than 10; heavy sleepers tend to have a higher temperature and shorter reaction times. Insomniacs need not worry about seeing furry worms, however. Not only do studies show they get more sleep than they actually think they do, but the loss of sleep is very rarely damaging—the body nearly always makes up for it.

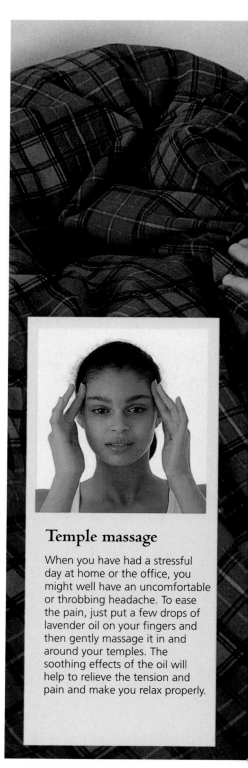

Temple massage

When you have had a stressful day at home or the office, you might well have an uncomfortable or throbbing headache. To ease the pain, just put a few drops of lavender oil on your fingers and then gently massage it in and around your temples. The soothing effects of the oil will help to relieve the tension and pain and make you relax properly.

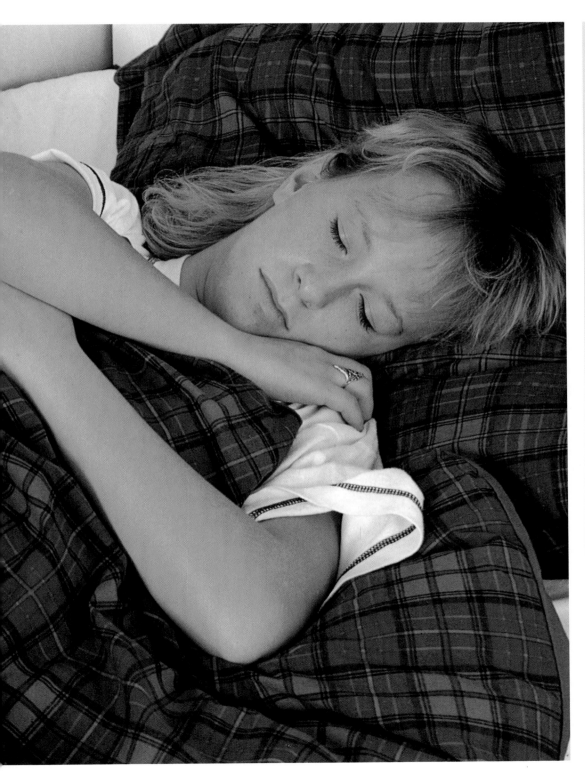

Most sleeping pills contain benzodiazepine, which is safe and effective but can lead to dependence, so try to find an alternative solution from the following:

● Drinking passiflora or valerian tea can help you to fall asleep, as can a few drops of lavender oil sprinkled on your pillow.

● The traditional bedtime warm milk and toast can be effective. Milk helps to produce calming opiates.

● Try to exercise every day. Besides making you tired it will reduce anxiety—a cause of insomnia.

● Make sure you have a firm mattress and a warm but well-ventilated room.

● The techniques of self-hypnosis can be used to encourage sleep.

● Try adjusting your body clock by going to bed later and getting up a bit later.

Delight the Senses

The sensory organs of the human body are our link with the outside world. Without our senses we would have no perception of anyone or anything. It is our senses—hearing, sight, smell, touch, and taste—that forge our development as individuals and within societies, allowing us to understand and measure the nuances of everyday experience.

One common idea about our senses is that they function as messengers, telling us what is going on around us—pointing out a car to the left, making us notice birds singing over there, and bringing to our attention the wonderful smell of baking bread. However, recent brain research shows that our senses are more sophisticated than that. Far from being passive receivers, they are actively involved in creating the world as we know it.

Our eyes, for instance, filter the tremendous amount of information that strikes them every second to produce the much smaller amount that the brain is able to process.

If our eyes and ears just operated like cameras and tape recorders we wouldn't be prey to illusions. These happen when essential working assumptions that the brain makes—bigger things are nearer, for instance—turn out not to be accurate.

Sensational scents

Each smell receptor is actually the far end of a group of brain cells making direct contact with the outside world. The other end is near the area of the brain connected with emotions and memory, which is why scents can have such a powerful effect. Most of us have experienced how smells can trigger a memory of things that happened in the past, of moments of great contentment, sorrow, or passion.

There is a long tradition of using scents and smells to change our moods and much current research involves using this ability to elicit particular responses from people. The Japanese, for example, have even managed to improve the performance of their work force by filtering the stimulating smell of lemon essential oil through the air-conditioning system in offices. Similarly, the smell of fresh coffee is suggested by real-estate agents to their clients as a means of encouraging buyers.

Using essential oils

Learn how to use the power of scent to create a relaxing or stimulating atmosphere in a room. There are several ways that you can enhance your environment aromatically:

1. Place a few drops of oil on a light bulb.
2. Place a few drops of oil on the wick of a candle before lighting it.
3. Put 6 to 7 drops of oil in a small bowl of warm water and then place it under or on a radiator.
4. An aroma diffuser or oil burner heats oils. Fill the pot with water and add 3 to 4 drops of your chosen oils, then light a candle under the pot to fill the room with fragrance (right).
5. Add oils to wood in an open fire or to water in an atomizer and spray the room.
6. A vaporizer can be used too. Add about 6 drops of oil.

Experiment with the following oil recipes to evoke the atmosphere you desire, whether to enhance or change your mood, or to set the scene for a special occasion.

Stimulating: Ylang-ylang, black pepper, and ginger
Euphoric: Clary sage, jasmine, and patchouli
Exotic: Ylang-ylang, sandalwood, and ginger
Luxurious: Rose, sandalwood, and ylang-ylang

- If you are irritable, anxious, or tired, try a mix of rose, neroli, and sandalwood to soothe you and lift the atmosphere around you. Another excellent mix for these symptoms is cedarwood and frankincense.
- Depression that comes from fear or despondency may respond to a mix of clary sage with bergamot or with frankincense and ylang-ylang.
- Lethargy and even grief may respond well to a frankincense and ylang-ylang mix.
- Your concentration may be considerably enhanced by combining peppermint and rosemary.

There are many other different combinations of oils that you can use.

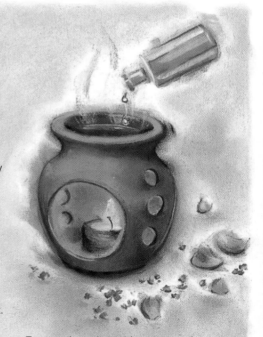

Try experimenting with a variety of mixes so you can find just the right scents to suit your moods.

Color your life

We are all in tune with the colors of our world, so much so that we all express our feelings in terms of color: We talk about being in the pink, feeling blue, seeing red, or being green with envy.

The psychological impact of color on our lives is deeper than we think. On the simplest level, we know that food manufacturers use color additives to boost our appetites and desire for their products, but color also has an effect on various other senses. If someone is shown a big box that is colored dark blue they will judge it to be much heavier than an identical box that is colored yellow. This is because yellow is a light, cheerful color, one we often dress children in, while dark blue is the color of contemplation and deep thought and is often used as a color for mourning. Further evidence comes from studies carried out on convalescing patients, who were found to recover better in rooms painted a soothing green or light blue. Also, violent prisoners will calm down if put in a pink room.

The colors you respond to can apparently tell you something about your own personality and state of mind; the colors of the rooms you live and work in or the clothes you wear can have a dramatic effect on your sense of well-being and on the reception you receive from those you meet. Once you know the effects colors can have on your emotional and physical well-being, you can use them to influence your life.

The psychology of color has been researched and studied by many people and the results have been used in psychiatric practices to reveal mental and emotional characteristics. One such test, the Color Reflection Reading, developed by Howard and Dorothy Sun, identifies a correlation between the colors chosen and particular traits of personality.

The Color Wheel

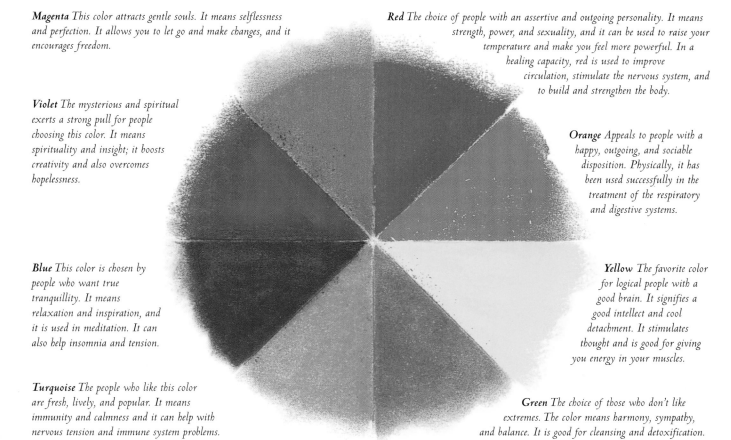

Magenta This color attracts gentle souls. It means selflessness and perfection. It allows you to let go and make changes, and it encourages freedom.

Violet The mysterious and spiritual exerts a strong pull for people choosing this color. It means spirituality and insight; it boosts creativity and also overcomes hopelessness.

Blue This color is chosen by people who want true tranquillity. It means relaxation and inspiration, and it is used in meditation. It can also help insomnia and tension.

Turquoise The people who like this color are fresh, lively, and popular. It means immunity and calmness and it can help with nervous tension and immune system problems.

Red The choice of people with an assertive and outgoing personality. It means strength, power, and sexuality, and it can be used to raise your temperature and make you feel more powerful. In a healing capacity, red is used to improve circulation, stimulate the nervous system, and to build and strengthen the body.

Orange Appeals to people with a happy, outgoing, and sociable disposition. Physically, it has been used successfully in the treatment of the respiratory and digestive systems.

Yellow The favorite color for logical people with a good brain. It signifies a good intellect and cool detachment. It stimulates thought and is good for giving you energy in your muscles.

Green The choice of those who don't like extremes. The color means harmony, sympathy, and balance. It is good for cleansing and detoxification.

> *"In truth, there is nothing like music to fill the moment with substance, whether it attunes the quiet mind to reverence and worship, or whether it makes the mobile senses dance in exultation."*
>
> GOETHE

Tips for developing your senses

Try out some of the following ideas to improve your sense perception:

● Listen to some favorite music with your eyes open, then closed, and notice the difference.

● Sit quietly with your eyes closed and rub a piece of material. Do it with your eyes open and notice any changes.

● Taste a food, again with your eyes open and then closed. See how one sense expands as another is eliminated.

● Sit and relax in a park, choose a letter of the alphabet and see how many things you can see that begin with that letter.

● Take a smell test with your eyes closed. Use aromatic oils, flowers, fruits, or vegetables and see what you can recognize.

Sound

Sound affects us on all levels: physical, emotional, mental, and spiritual. Hearing is probably the first sense that develops. The baby in the womb can hear its mother's heartbeat and later the sounds of the world outside, perceiving the world with its hearing before any other sense. At death, hearing is usually the last human sense to go.

One U.S. study found that one of the most powerful ways of changing a person's mood is with music. It was found to be comparable with techniques recommended by the medical profession, such as exercise and some forms of therapy, both for energizing and also for inducing a calm state of mind.

Music also seems to help in organizing the brain. Some research shows that children develop their abstract reasoning abilities more quickly if they have had early musical training. It has also been used for centuries to help soldiers on the march and workers to keep up a rhythm. In fact, African-American music originated in the songs sung by gangs of slaves at work in the fields.

The use of music and sound for healing goes back to ancient times. The mystery schools in the ancient temples of Egypt, Greece, and Rome considered vibration one of the fundamental forces in the universe. Specific tones and chants have been used for years to alter a person's state of consciousness and to heal the mind and body. Many Eastern cultures use mantras and chanting to connect the human experience to the divine.

A growing number of healers and health practitioners believe that specific sounds can affect the body and relieve pain. The idea is that every organ and even every cell has its own natural rate of vibration. Poor health may be the result of changes in these natural rates, which can be restored by bathing a changed area with particular sounds.

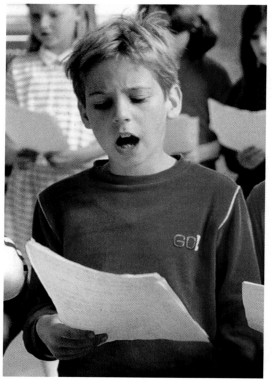

Singing is a very enjoyable experience in which all our emotions can be expressed. Being part of a choir and singing Christmas carols or hymns can be very uplifting.

Sing your stress away

There is nothing like a good sing-along to release pent-up anxiety and stress. Singing not only is a joy in its own right but is an effective way of releasing tension and increasing creativity in your life. Singing is a natural means of communication. It also improves the resonance, power, and flexibility of your speaking as well as your singing voice. Your breathing becomes deeper, and you can reduce stress and tension.

Have you ever noticed how much better you feel after you have sung along with the radio? There are physiological reasons for these changes–an increased respiratory movement stimulates the circulatory system feeding the brain and other organs.

Try the "Ahh" exercise to release stress. Stand with feet apart, shoulders relaxed with arms at your sides, and take a deep breath, inhaling through your nose. Open your mouth wide and exhale as you say "Ahhh . . ."–long, loud, and down to deep, low tones until you have exhaled completely. Repeat three times.

Touch

The importance of the power of touch in our lives is all too frequently ignored or forgotten. Hugging and expressing our feelings of love and affection through touch has become a neglected art in our busy, modern, stress-filled lives. Cuddles and hugs are expressions of affection that many people fail to feel comfortable with, not realizing that touch might hold the key to their well-being and that of their family.

Earlier this century, an American researcher named Harlow showed how touch is essential for normal human development and for mental and emotional well-being. Research showed that baby monkeys who were deprived of maternal tactile interaction became withdrawn, neurotic, and even psychotic, unable to relate to the other monkeys. Humans have similarities to monkeys and touch is no less important to us.

Touching is a universal language that everyone uses to communicate. Unconsciously or consciously, we need to show the way we feel about ourselves and about one another. It can mean so much to us. We use touch to show intimacy and closeness—with our partner, our children, family, and close friends. We also use touch to show approval, how much we care, friendship, and love.

Recent studies in this country have shown that premature babies who are stroked and cuddled from the moment they are born have far fewer nonbreathing periods, gain weight, and thrive far faster than those babies who have received little or no physical contact.

But studies are not needed to tell us what every mother knows from experience—that touching and holding soothes and reassures a child more effectively than anything else, especially if the child has become upset and frightened.

It is a well-established fact that people who have been neglected by their parents and starved for affection may have serious emotional and physical problems later in life. Touching someone is so simple, and yet it can become so difficult, if it is not a habit learned in the formative years.

Touching and being touched makes us feel good or, at the least, better. The power of massage to relieve stress and tension and generally make us feel better has been known for centuries. The close intimacy of massaging a loved one can also bring a further warmth and depth to a relationship. Without enough touch in our lives we can become stunted, withdrawn, and alienated. True, the amount of touching between people is a function of culture and how well people know each other, but everyone is responsive to touch. In times of trouble and severe emotional trauma, a hug can be very reassuring and healing.

Some experts believe that much of the pleasures we experience when kissing or making love comes down to the pleasure of being touched, held, and stroked. Other interesting studies have shown how the heart rates of people stroking their pets is lowered, only to rise again when they stop stroking the animal. There is no doubting the deep power of touch to improve the state of our minds and therefore our bodies.

By touching the people close to you more often you will enhance and increase your general well-being.

Cuddling or stroking a loved pet can be very reassuring for people of all ages, and can help improve general well-being.

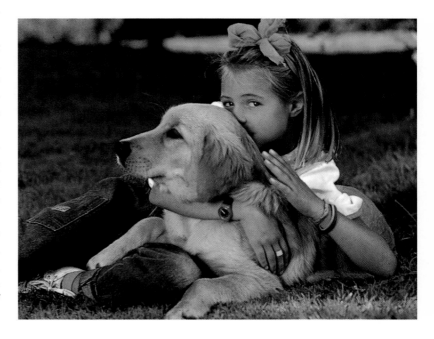

Creating a Tranquil Environment

Who can deny the sense of peace and harmony you feel when you walk into a room that successfully surrounds you with its tranquil and balanced atmosphere? You may look around the room and wonder just exactly what it is that makes it work. Why do you feel so good in this space? It can be a room at home, at someone else's house, or at work. There are probably a number of factors that contribute to creating a tranquil and uplifting environment.

First, rooms that use all, or almost all, natural materials and fibers will feel healthier because they *are* healthier. Synthetic carpets and upholstery, foam insulation, and any number of other synthetic materials emit formaldehyde, which can cause adverse reactions in some people. Varnishes, lacquers, and glues, often used in the manufacture of furniture, contain trichloroethylene, which can irritate the eyes, skin, and sinuses and cause headaches. Practical solutions include having natural wood floors, buying natural fiber upholstery, rugs, and curtains, especially if you or members of your family are allergy-sensitive or suffer from asthma.

Good ventilation and airflow are also very important. Another way of creating a happy, healthy environment in which to live and work is to share your space with some plants. These are not just for decoration, although the sight of greenery is known to reduce stress, but also for reducing the pollution in any room and adding moisture to the air. The benefit of indoor plants is even recognized by NASA, the space agency, which makes sure some plants are always included in their spacecraft.

Key to creating a tranquil bedroom

To create a restful, relaxing environment, choose a bedroom away from any intrusive exterior sounds, such as traffic noise, and if possible away from the hustle and bustle of the rest of the house. Decorate the room with natural fabrics in colors that are restful to the eye. Wooden floors create a sense of peace and provide a healthier environment by being easy to dust and clean. A natural-fiber rug in a soothing color can add to the mellow mood. Plants not only help reduce environmental pollution but they perfume the air, assisting in relaxation. Reducing clutter helps promote a more restful space, as does resolving not to do anything associated with work in your special room.

The color of rooms

Color experts claim that if you change the color of your room you can change your life—and we have all experienced the positive and uplifting effect of a new paint color on the walls.

We are much more influenced by the colors around us than we realize and we should endeavor to find the shade that makes us feel the most relaxed in order to restore a little balance to our lives. Paler blues and greens are healing, balancing colors that are good for bedrooms, while the warm colors of yellow, orange, and peach are ideal for kitchens and front doors where people come together to communicate. Alternately, you may respond more to the darker, deeper, rich

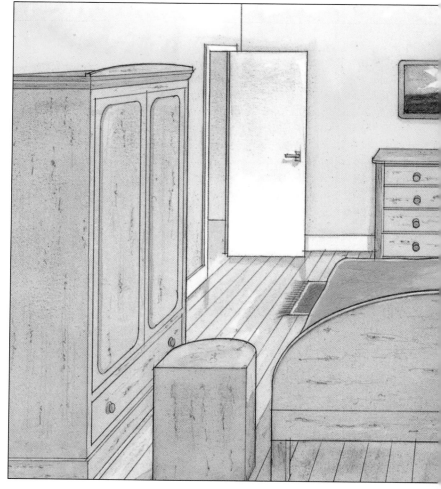

colors like red and purple. If the color works for you, it works–that's the key. Color perception and favorite colors are very personal, but there are some guidelines to follow, according to the color experts. For example, if you are a very energetic, overstimulated, passionate, or emotional person, try to cool your environment with blues, greens, lilacs, and pinks. However, if you are too relaxed for work and need stimulation, try using bold reds, oranges, and yellows as part of your interior design. Another color rule is to avoid using too much of any one color. Instead, try to match complementary colors to achieve the right balance and variety.

Some complementary combinations:
• blue and yellow • violet and yellow • pink and green • magenta and green • red and turquoise • orange and blue • yellow and gray.

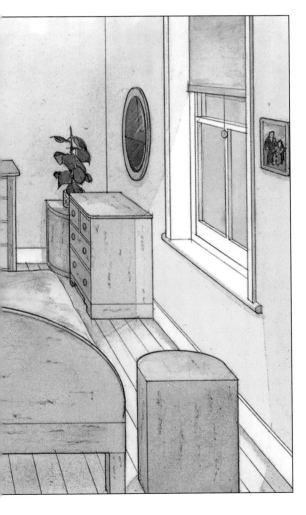

Feng Shui

Feng Shui is the ancient Chinese art of placement and energy flow. The Chinese believe energy moves through the environment in the same way it does through the body: It can flow freely and smoothly or it can become blocked and stuck, causing imbalance, and in severe cases, illness.

Feng Shui is said to work on a room or a building in the same way that acupuncture works on the body: It balances the energies and gets them flowing freely again. This is taken so seriously in China that most architects and owners of buildings employ a Feng Shui expert to give a clean bill of health to their new building projects.

In Feng Shui, different spaces in a room have different functions, and this also applies to your entire home. Experts use a map, the ba-gua, that plots eight different areas in your home related to career, marriage, children, family, fame, wealth, knowledge, and helpful people in your life.

An increasing number of people in the West are adopting the concepts of Feng Shui and are now considering their living and working spaces in a new light, gaining a greater understanding of the various effects rooms and the placement of furniture can have on us and our lives.

By the careful placing of objects, such as plants and mirrors, you can block the flow of bad Feng Shui, while moving furniture to more favorable sites can open up good Feng Shui energy channels, known as ch'i. Clutter in a room can deflect the flow of ch'i. Instead, hang pictures or ornaments on the wall. An aquarium of fish will also help the flow of ch'i within your home.

One of the most important areas of your living room is the wealth point, which is situated on the top left-hand corner of the room as you enter. A door or doorway under this point will encourage your money to disappear. If this is the case, grow a plant with large, rounded leaves there. This will reflect the increase in your income—the larger the plant, the larger the increase!

Feng Shui at home

Apply some of the Feng Shui techniques to your own home, not only to improve the environment and atmosphere but also your general health and well-being.

• "Spring clean" regularly. In other words, clear out all the clutter in your home.

• Give or throw away items you don't need.

• Keep your rooms tidy, clean, and bright.

• Keep houseplants well placed and nurtured to keep the air clean and the room's energy alive.

• The leaves of plants should be rounded.

• Keep plants near or on electronic equipment to counteract negative electromagnetic effects.

• Use mirrors to enhance and expand the energy of a room.

• Carefully sited wind chimes can bring you good luck, particularly in financial matters.

Living in the Present

Change is inevitable in all our lives. Some changes we welcome, others we find challenging or a cause for concern. Life is often filled with regrets, recriminations, dissatisfaction, and sorrow. But does it need to be? Our attitude toward the world directly affects what happens in our lives. Those with a positive attitude grasp each day as it comes, welcoming the challenges, accepting the various happy or sad, difficult or easy moments. They acknowledge life for what it is—the most precious gift we have. Thinking that today is the start of your life can give you a much more positive outlook on the rest of your life.

Living in the present does not mean that we should give up all our memories or never look to the future, but it does mean paying more attention to what is happening and how we feel, think, and act right now. Sometimes we can be so busy and so convoluted in our approach to everyday life that we can miss the simple beauty and joy of present pleasures. We must learn not to take our daily lives too much for granted.

Living in the present means being a whole person. If you savor the life within and around you, the vitality and potential of the present, you will learn to let go of the negative habits that keep you dwelling on the past or thinking "everything would be all right if only. . . ." You will leave behind beliefs and conditioning that have thrown shadows across your existence.

If we stop to really consider our lives and the many influences, including family, friends, and events, that have shaped us, we come to realize that the only constant in life is change. Furthermore, we come to realize that most things are beyond our control. The only true control we have is over our thoughts, ideas, beliefs, and attitudes. At the end of the day, whether you are happy or sad in your life is up to you. You make that decision because you decide whether to project either a positive or negative attitude.

You need to remember that whatever challenge life presents, you will be able to cope. With positive energy and application you will be successful.

Many people say that the key to real happiness lies within our own minds, not in the outside world. Do not always look to the future; enjoy the journey to your goals, as well as achieving the goals themselves. Be ever mindful of the present, appreciate the opportunities that come your way, enjoy your leisure time—and you will really make the most of your life.

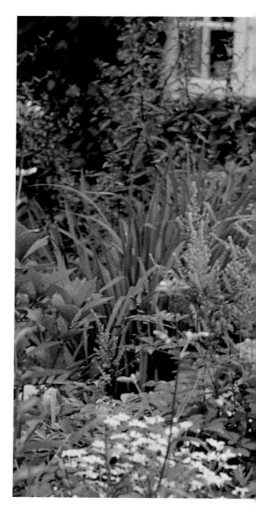

Work and play

One of the important keys to a happy life is a balanced approach to work and play. It is very important for your physical, mental, and emotional well-being to make time for pleasurable pursuits. Only a very few people have the good fortune to make a living from doing what they like best. For the rest of us, we must do our best to create the time and space to indulge our special needs, after time spent with family and friends.

It makes no difference what your special interest is: It could be cooking, gardening, reading, or playing golf. What does matter is that you recognize what you love to do and do it!

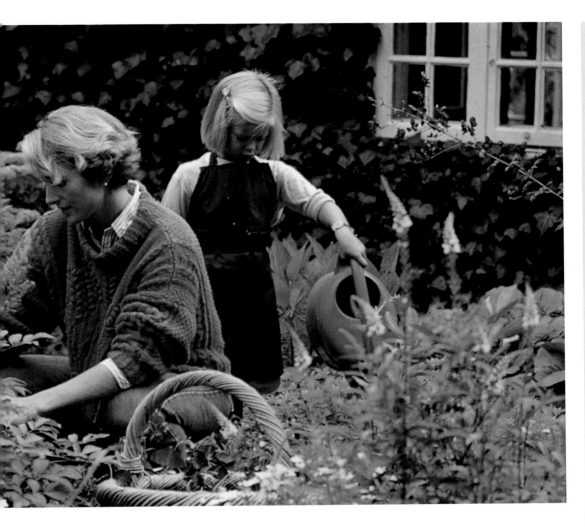

Tips for recharging

If you are feeling stressed and don't have enough time to yourself, here are some positive things you can do to help you feel better:

● Be kind to yourself on a regular basis. Do what you need to do to change a negative self-image.

● Learn and practice accepting and forgiving yourself more—nobody expects you to be perfect.

● Take some time each day or every other day to do some deep-breathing exercises.

● Create some personal space within your immediate environment. Spend 15 to 30 minutes meditating every day in that space.

● Have a massage, facial, or other beauty treatment to revive you.

● Spend as much time as possible doing the things you love most. Just do the things you want to do.

Making time for a special time

Life today is incredibly pressurized with everyone working at a furious pace to earn a living and run busy households. But all of us need time alone, so try to take 30 to 60 minutes each day to take stock of yourself and to give yourself some pampered relaxation. Do whatever works best for you to recharge your batteries, get in touch with yourself, and recognize your true value. Through making the effort to take time out just for you, you can improve your relationship with your partner, your lifestyle, and your overall quality of life.

The world is your oyster and your life is literally what you make it. It is worth remembering the words of Kabat-Zinn, who said, "Mindfulness is a road map to our radiant selves, not to the gold of a childhood innocence already past but to that of a fully developed adult. It is a way of walking along the path of life and being in harmony with things as they are."

Gardening is one of the most therapeutic and satisfying hobbies that can be done by anyone at a time to suit them. It is even used as a therapy for brain-damaged people because it is very rewarding and helps to restore different abilities, including coordination.

Acknowledgments

The publisher thanks the photographers for their kind permission to reproduce the following photographs in this book:

13 Explorer/P Royer; 20 Marie Claire Idées/Chabaneix/Chabaneix/Paillard; 25 Collections/Sandra Lousada; 26 Jerrican/Perlstein; 27 Camera Press/Box Office; 28 Collections/Anthea Sieveking; 68 Collections/Sandra Lousada; 70 M C Picture Library/Bill Petch; 73 Marie Claire Idées/Christian Moser; 76–77 Collections/Sandra Lousada; 78 Robert Harding Picture Library/Michelle Garrett; 79 S & O Mathews; 84 The Image Bank/Carol Kohen; 86–87 Marie Claire/Chatelain; 90 Diaf/Dannic; 91 Tony Stone Images/Joe Cornish; 93 The Image Bank/G & M David de Lossy; 94–95 Rex Features; 96 Jerrican/Guignard; 97 Jerrican/Perlstein; 114 Zefa; 118 Tony Stone Images/Howard Grey; 119 Explorer/A Essarton; 120–121 The Image Bank; 126 Stephen P Huyler; 127 Graham Harrison; 128 Explorer/F Chazott; 129 Marie Claire Idees/Yoichiro Sato/Martine Paillard; 130 Collections/Sandra Lousada; 130–131 Explorer/Ph Roy; 134 Collections/Sandra Lousada; 135 Explorer/A Essartons; 138–139 The Image Bank/Werner Bokelberg.

The following photographs were taken by Sandra Lousada:
4–11, 14–19, 21–23, 30, 48, 66, 72, 74–75, 80–81, 85, 88, 98–110, 122–125.

The following photographs were taken by Carl Warner:
43–47, 50–65

The editors gratefully acknowledge Peter Simester, Philip and Eleanor Schwartz, Jane Silk, Jane Alexander, Jennifer Dodd, Pierre Jean Cousins, Geraldine Rich, Michael Skipwith, Chris James, Eddie and Debbie Shapiro, James South, Howard and Dorothy Sun, Jane Rappeport, Alexander Galitzine, Juliet Gellatley, and Alex and Martina Lowson for their help and support.

Further Reading

Healthy Bones Nancy Appleton (Avery 1991)
Ageless Body, Timeless Mind Deepak Chopra (Health & Healing 1993)
You Can Heal Your Life Louise L. Hay (Eden Grove Editions 1984)
The BMA Complete Family Health Encyclopedia (Dorling Kindersley)
Family Guide to Alternative Medicine (Reader's Digest)
A New Model for Health and Disease George Vithoulkas (Health and Habitat 1991)
Choosing Health Intentionally Xandria Williams (Letts 1990)
Super Foods Michael van Stratten & Barbara Griggs (Dorling Kindersley)
Food Combining for Health Doris Grant & Jean Joice (Thorsons 1984)
The Food Combining Diet (Thorsons 1993)
The Bristol Diet Dr Alec Forbes (Century Arrow)
Fresh Vegetable & Fruit Juices: What's Missing in Your Diet N.W. Walker (Norwalk Press, USA)
Lifeforce Julie Chrystyn (Smith Gryphon 1994)
Royal Jelly: The New Guide to Nature's Richest Health Food Irene Stein (Thorsons 1989)
Your Body is Your Best Doctor Melvin E. Page & H. Leon Abrams (Keats 1972)
The Family Guide to Homeopathy Dr Andrew Lockie (Elm Tree Books 1989)
Aromatherapy for Women Maggie Tisserand (Thorsons 1985)
Better Health Through Natural Healing Ross Trattler (Thorsons 1985)
Alternative Dictionary of Symptoms & Cures Dr Caroline M. Shreeve (Century)
The Book of Yoga Lucy Lidell (Gaia)
The Bodymind Workbook Debbie Shapiro (Element 1990)
Out of Your Mind–The Only Place To Be Eddie & Debbie Shapiro (Element 1992)
Stress Busters Robert Holden (Thorsons)
Relax: Dealing with Stress Murray Watts & Prof. Cary L. Cooper (BBC Books)
A Time for Healing Eddie & Debbie Shapiro (Piatkus 1994)
The Tao of Health, Sex and Longevity Daniel Reid (Simon & Schuster 1989)
Colour Your Life Howard & Dorothy Sun (Piatkus)
Creating Sacred Space with Feng Shui Karen Kingston (Piatkus 1996)
Healing Sounds: The Power of Harmonics Jonathon Goldman (Element 1992)

GENERAL

American Board of Medical Specialties
1007 Church Street, Suite 404
Evanston, IL 60201
phone: (800) 776-CERT
(Will tell you if your physician is board certified.)

American Holistic Medical Association (AHMA)
Suite 201
4101 Lake Boone Trail
Raleigh, NC 27607
fax: (919) 787-4916
(Will provide national referral directory for a fee; send written request.)

Centers for Disease Control and Prevention
1600 Clifton Road, NE
Atlanta, GA 30333
phone: (404) 639-3311

National Library of Medicine
8600 Rockville Pike
Bethesda, MD 20894
phone: (301) 496-6095
telnet for access to on-line catalog: locator.nlm.nih.gov
[Login as "locator".]
www: http://www.nlm.nih.gov/
(Medical and scientific books and journals.)

ACUPUNCTURE AND CHINESE MEDICINE

National Acupuncture and Oriental Medicine Alliance
PO Box 77511
Seattle, WA 98177-0531
phone: (206) 524-3511
fax: (206) 728-4841
E-mail:
76143.2061@compuserve.com

National Commission for the Certification of Acupuncturists
PO Box 97075
Washington, DC 20090-7075
phone: (202) 232-1404
fax: (202) 462-6157
(Does not give referrals; will send list of certified acupuncturists for a fee.)

AGING

National Institute on Aging
Information Center
PO Box 8057
Gaithersburg, MD 20898-8057
phone: (800) 222-2225
fax: (301) 589-3014
E-mail: niainfo@access.digex.net

AYURVEDIC MEDICINE

Ayurvedic Institute
11311 Menaul NE, Suite A
Albuquerque, NM 87112
phone: (505) 291-9698

BODY WORK

American Massage Therapy Association
820 Davis Street, Suite 100
Evanston, IL 60201-4444
phone: (708) 864-0123
fax: (708) 864-1178

Aston-Patterning
PO Box 3568
Incline Village, NV 89450-3568
phone: (702) 831-8228
fax: (702) 831-8955
E-mail: astonpat@aol.com

Feldenkrais Guild
PO Box 489
Albany, OR 97321
phone: (800) 775-2118

International Institute of Reflexology
PO Box 12462
St. Petersburg, FL 33733
phone: (813) 343-4811

North American Society of Teachers of the Alexander Technique
PO Box 517
Urbana, IL 61801
phone: (800) 473-0620

Rolf Institute of Structural Integration
205 Canyon Boulevard
Boulder, CO 80302
phone: (303) 449-5903;
(800) 530-8875
fax: (303) 449-5978
E-mail: rolfinst@aol.com

CANCER

American Cancer Society
1599 Clifton Road, NE
Atlanta, GA 30329-4251
phone: (800) ACS-2345
fax: (404) 325-2217
www:http://www.cancer.org/

CancerCare
1180 Avenue of the Americas
New York, NY 10036
phone: (212) 302-2400;
(800) 813-HOPE
fax: (212) 719-0263

National Alliance of Breast Cancer Organizations (NABCO)
9 E. 37th Street, 10th Floor
New York, NY 10016
phone: (212) 719-0154
fax: (212) 689-1213
E-mail: nabcoinfo@aol.com

National Cancer Institute's Cancer Information Service
phone: (800) 4CANCER

Skin Cancer Foundation
PO Box 561
New York, NY 10156

phone: (212) 725-5176;
(800) SKIN490
fax: (212) 725-5751

CHILDREN'S HEALTH

American Academy of Pediatrics
PO Box 927
Elk Grove Village, IL 60009-0927
(Send self-addressed, stamped business envelope with information request.)

CHIROPRACTIC

American Chiropractic Association
1701 Clarendon Boulevard
Arlington, VA 22209
phone: (703) 276-8800
fax: (703) 243-2593
E-mail: merchiro@aol.com

DENTAL PROBLEMS

American Dental Association
211 E. Chicago Avenue
Chicago, IL 60611
www: http://www.ada.org/

DIGESTION/ GASTROINTESTINAL PROBLEMS

Celiac Sprue Association, USA
PO Box 31700
Omaha, NE 68131
phone: (402) 558-0600
fax: (402) 558-1347

Crohn's & Colitis Foundation of America
386 Park Avenue South
New York, NY 10016-8804
phone: (212) 685-3440;
(800) 932-2423
fax: (212) 779-4098
E-mail: mhda37b@prodigy.com

National Digestive Diseases Information Clearinghouse
2 Information Way
Bethesda, MD 20892-3570
fax: (301) 907-8906

EAR, NOSE, AND THROAT PROBLEMS

American Academy of Otolaryngology-Head and Neck Surgery
1 Prince Street
Alexandria, VA 22314
phone: (703) 836-4444
TTY/TDD: (703) 519-1585
fax: (703) 683-5100

American Tinnitus Association
PO Box 5
Portland, OR 97207-0005
phone: (503) 248-9985
fax: (503) 248-0024

ENDOCRINE PROBLEMS

American Diabetes Association (ADA)
1660 Duke Street
Alexandria, VA 22314
phone: (800) DIABETES
(342-2383)
www: http://www.diabetes.org/

National Diabetes Information Clearinghouse (NDIC)
1 Information Way
Bethesda, MD 20892-3560
fax: (301) 907-8906

Thyroid Foundation of America, Inc.
Ruth Sleeper Hall, RSL 350
40 Parkman Street
Boston, MA 02114
phone: (617) 726-8500;
(800) 832-8321
fax: (617) 726-4136

ENVIRONMENTAL ILLNESS

American Academy of Environmental Medicine
4510 W. 89th Street, Suite 110
Prairie Village, KS 66207
phone: (913) 642-6062
fax: (913) 341-6912
E-mail:
71072.2356@compuserve.com
www:
http://www.netplace.net/aaem/

EYE PROBLEMS

American Academy of Ophthalmology
PO Box 7424
San Francisco, CA 94120-7424
phone: (415) 561-8500
fax: (415) 561-8567
E-mail: webmaster@eyenet.org
www: http://www.eyenet.org/

National Eye Institute
2020 Vision Place
Bethesda, MD 20892-3655
phone: (301) 496-5248
fax: (301) 402-1065
E-mail: 2020@b31.nei.nih.gov

FITNESS

American Council on Exercise
5820 Oberlin Drive, Suite 102
San Diego, CA 92121-3787
phone: (619) 535-8227
FITNESS HOTLINE: (800) 529-8227
fax: (619) 535-1778

HEART AND CIRCULATORY PROBLEMS

American Board of Chelation Therapy
1407B N. Wells Street
Chicago, IL 60610
phone: (800) 356-2228
(For information or referrals, send a self-addressed, stamped envelope.)

American Heart Association
7272 Greenville Avenue
Dallas, TX 75231-4596
phone: (214) 373-6300;
(800) AHA-USA1
fax: (214) 706-1341
www: http://www.amhrt.org/

National Heart, Lung, and Blood Institute Information Center
PO Box 30105
Bethesda, MD 20824-0105
phone: (800) 575-WELL
fax: (301) 251-1223
E-mail: hlbiic@DGS.dgsys.com

HEMATOLIGICAL/HEPATOLO GICAL

American Liver Foundation
1425 Pompton Avenue
Cedar Grove, NJ 07009
phone: (201) 256-2550;
(800) 223-0179
fax: (201) 256-3214

The Sickle Cell Disease Association of America
200 Corporate Pointe,
Suite 495
Culver City, CA 90230-7633
phone: (310) 216-6363;
(800) 421-8453
fax: (310) 215-3722

HERBS

Herb Research Foundation
1007 Pearl Street, Suite 200
Boulder, CO 80302
phone: (800) 748-2617

HOMEOPATHY

International Foundation for Homeopathy
2366 Eastlake Avenue East,
Suite 329
Seattle, WA 98102
phone: (206) 324-8230

National Center for Homeopathy
801 N. Fairfax Street, Suite 306
Alexandria, VA 22314
phone: (703) 548-7790
fax: (703) 548-7792

IMMUNE DISORDERS

AIDS Clinical Trials Information Service (ACTIS)
PO Box 6421
Rockville, MD 20850
phone: (800) TRIALS-A
TTY/TDD: (800) 243-7012
fax: (301) 738-6616

American Academy of Allergy, Asthma & Immunology
611 E. Wells Street
Milwaukee, WI 53202
phone: (800) 822-2762

CDC National AIDS
Clearinghouse
PO Box 6003
Rockville, MD 20849-6003
phone: (301) 217-0023
(800) 458-5231
TTY/TDD: (800) 243-7012
fax: (301) 738-6616
E-mail:
aidsinfo@cdcnac.aspensys.com
www:
http://cdcnac.aspensys.com:86/

CDC National HIV/AIDS
Hotline
phone: (800) 342-AIDS (2437)
Spanish access: (800) 344-
SIDA (7432)
TTY/TDD: (800) AIDSTTY
(243-7889)

CFIDS Association of America
PO Box 220398
Charlotte, NC 28222-0398
phone: (800) 442-3437
fax: (704) 365-9755
(Chronic fatigue and immune
dysfunction syndromes.)

Lupus Foundation of America
4 Research Place, Suite 180
Rockville, MD 20850-3226
phone: (301) 670-9292;
(800) 558-0121
Spanish access: (800) 558-0231
fax: (301) 670-9486

National Institute of Allergy
and Infectious Diseases
Office of Communications
Building 31, Room 7A-50
31 Center Drive, MSC 2520
Bethesda, MD 20892-2520

LUNG DISEASE
American Lung Association
1740 Broadway
New York, NY 10019-4374
phone: (212) 315-8700;
(800) LUNG-USA
fax: (212) 265-5642
E-mail: info@lungusa.org

MAGNETIC FIELD THERAPY
Bio-Electro-Magnetics
Institute (BEMI)
2490 West Moana Lane
Reno, NV 89509-7801
phone: (702) 827-9099
E-mail: johnz@scs.unr.edu

MENTAL HEALTH
American Psychiatric
Association
Division of Public Affairs
1400 K Street, NW
Washington, DC 20005
phone: (202) 682-6220
fax: (202) 682-6255
E-mail: paffairs@psych.org

Children and Adults with
Attention Deficit Disorders
(CH.A.D.D.)
499 Northwest 70th Avenue,
Suite 101
Plantation, FL 33317
phone: (305) 587-3700;
(800) 233-4050
fax: (305) 587-4599
E-mail: info@chadd.org
www: http://www.chadd.org/

Depression & Related
Affective Disorders
Association (DRADA)
Meyer 3-181
600 North Wolfe Street
Baltimore, MD 21287-7381
phone: (410) 955-4647
fax: (410) 614-3241

National Institute of
Mental Health
Information Resources and
Inquiries 5600 Fishers Lane,
Room 7C-02
Rockville, MD 20857

National Mental Health
Association (NMHA)
Information Center, 30
1021 Prince Street
Alexandria, VA 22314-2971
phone: (703) 684-7722;
(800) 969-NMHA
fax: (703) 684-5968

MIND-BODY MEDICINE
Association for Applied
Psychophysiology and
Biofeedback
10200 W. 44th Avenue
Suite 304
Wheat Ridge, CO 80033-2840
fax: (303) 422-8894
E-mail: 5686814@mcimail.com
(Send a self-addressed,
stamped envelope for further
information or a list of
physicians in your area.)

MUSCULOSKELETAL
PROBLEMS
Arthritis Foundation
PO Box 7669
Atlanta, GA 30357
phone: (800) 283-7800
fax: (404) 872-0457
E-mail: info@arthritis.org

National Osteoporosis
Foundation
1150 17th Street, NW
Suite 500
Washington, DC 20036
phone: (800) 223-9994
www: http://www.nof.org/

Scoliosis Association, Inc.
PO Box 811705
Boca Raton, FL 33481-1705
phone: (800) 800-0669

NATUROPATHIC MEDICINE
American Association
of Naturopathic Physicians
2366 Eastlake Avenue East,
Suite 322
Seattle, WA 98102
phone: (206) 323-7610
fax: (206) 323-7612

NEUROLOGICAL PROBLEMS
Alzheimer's Association
919 N. Michigan Avenue,
Suite 1000
Chicago, IL 60611-1676
phone: (312) 335-8700;
(800) 272-3900
fax: (312) 335-1110
www: http://www.alz.org/

American Parkinson
Disease Association
1250 Hylan Boulevard
Suite 4B
Staten Island, NY 10305
phone: (718) 981-8001;
(800) 223-2732
fax: (718) 981-4399

The Amyotrophic Lateral
Sclerosis Association
National Office
21021 Ventura Boulevard,
Suite 321
Woodland Hills, CA 91364
phone: (818) 340-7500;
(800) 782-4747
fax: (818) 340-2060

The Epilepsy Foundation of
America
4351 Garden City Drive
Landover, MD 20785
phone: (301) 459-3700
E-mail: postmaster@efa.org

The Multiple Sclerosis
Foundation
6350 N. Andrews Avenue
Ft. Lauderdale, FL 33309
phone: (800) 441-7055

National Headache
Foundation
428 West St. James Place,
2nd Floor
Chicago, IL 60614
phone: (800) 843-2256

Parkinson's Disease
Foundation (PDF)
710 W. 168th Street
New York, NY 10032
phone: (212) 923-4700;
(800) 457-6676
fax: (212) 923-4778
E-mail: pdf cpmc@aol.com

NUTRITION AND DIET
American Dietetic Association
National Center for Nutrition
and Dietetics
216 W. Jackson Boulevard,

Suite 800
Chicago, IL 60606
ADA's Consumer Nutrition
Hotline: (800) 366-1655

OSTEOPATHY
American Osteopathic
Association
142 East Ontario Street
Chicago, IL 60611
phone: (800) 621-1773 x7401

SEXUAL HEALTH
CDC's National STD Hotline
(800) 227-8922
8 am-11 pm EST, M-F

Couple to Couple League
International, Inc.
PO Box 111184
Cincinnati, OH 45211-1184
phone: (513) 471-2000
fax: (513) 557-2449
(Natural family planning.)

Impotence Institute of
America
10400 Little Patuxent Parkway
Suite 485
Columbia, MD 21044-3502
phone: (410) 715-9605;
(800) 669-1603
fax: (410) 715-9609

Planned Parenthood
Federation
of America, Inc.
810 Seventh Avenue
New York, NY 10019
phone: (212) 541-7800;
(800) 669-0156 for
publications
fax: (212) 245-1845

SKIN
American Academy of
Dermatology
PO Box 4014
Schaumburg, IL 60168-4014
phone: (708) 330-0230
fax: (708) 330-0050
www: http://www.derm-
infonet.com/

SUBSTANCE ABUSE
Alcoholics Anonymous
PO Box 459
Grand Central Station
New York, NY 10163
phone: (212) 870-3400

Narcotics Anonymous
World Service Office
PO Box 9999
Van Nuys, CA 91409
phone: (818) 773-9999
fax: (818) 700-0700

National Institute on Alcohol
Abuse and Alcoholism
6000 Executive Boulevard
Willco Building

Bethesda, MD 20892-7003
phone: (301) 443-3860
fax: (301) 443-6077

URINARY TRACT PROBLEMS
National Kidney and Urologic
Diseases Information
Clearinghouse
3 Information Way
Bethesda, MD 20892-3580
fax: (301) 907-8906

National Kidney
Foundation, Inc.
30 E. 33rd Street, 11th Floor
New York, NY 10016
phone: (212) 889-2210;
(800) 622-9010
fax: (212) 689-9261

WOMEN'S HEALTH
American College of
Obstetricians and Gynecol-
ogists, Resource Center
409 12th Street, SW
Washington, DC 20024
(For patient education
brochures, send a self-
addressed, stamped business
envelope and specify topic of
interest.)

Human Development
Resource Council, Inc.
3941 Holcomb Bridge Road,
Suite 300
Norcross, GA 30092
phone: (770) 447-1598
fax: (770) 447-0759

National Women's Health
Network
514 10th Street, NW, Suite 400
Washington, DC 20004
phone: (202) 628-7814

YOGA
International Association
of Yoga Therapists
109 Hillside Avenue
Mill Valley, CA 94941
phone: (415) 383-4587
fax: (415) 381-0876
E-mail: yoganet@aol.com
(Send self-addressed, stamped
envelope for an educational
brochure on finding a yoga
teacher.)

MISCELLANEOUS
American Academy of
Neural Therapy
539 Harkle Road, Suite D
Santa Fe, NM 87505
phone: (505) 988-3086

American Apitherapy Society
PO Box 54
Hartland Four Corners, VT
05049
phone: (800) 823-3460

Index